Study and Review Guide to accompany

ANATOMY & PHYSIOLOGY

Sixth Edition

Gary A. Thibodeau
Kevin T. Patton

Written by: Linda Swisher, RN, EdD

MOSBY

ELSEVIER

11830 Westline Industrial Drive
St. Louis, Missouri 63146

Study Guide to accompany
Anatomy & Physiology, Sixth Edition

ISBN-13: 978-0-323-03723-5
ISBN-10: 0-323-03723-2

Notice

Knowledge and best practice in this field are constantly changing. As new research and experience broaden our knowledge, changes in practice, treatment and drug therapy may become necessary or appropriate. Readers are advised to check the most current information provided (i) on procedures featured or (ii) by the manufacturer of each product to be administered, to verify the recommended dose or formula, the method and duration of administration, and contraindications. It is the responsibility of the practitioner, relying on their own experience and knowledge of the patient, to make diagnoses, to determine dosages and the best treatment for each individual patient, and to take all appropriate safety precautions. To the fullest extent of the law, neither the Publisher nor the Authors assumes any liability for any injury and/or damage to persons or property arising out or related to any use of the material contained in this book.

The Publisher

ISBN-13: 978-0-323-03723-5
ISBN-10: 0-323-03723-2

Executive Editor: Thomas J. Wilhelm
Managing Editor: Jeff Downing
Associate Developmental Editor: Jennifer Stoces
Publishing Services Manager: Deborah L. Vogel
Senior Project Manager: Steve Ramay
Design Manager: Mark Oberkrom

Printed in the United States of America

Last digit is the print number: 9 8 7 6 5 4 3 2 1

Working together to grow
libraries in developing countries

www.elsevier.com | www.bookaid.org | www.sabre.org

ELSEVIER   BOOK AID International   Sabre Foundation

Introduction

This *Study and Review Guide to accompany Anatomy and Physiology, sixth* edition, is designed to help you be successful in learning anatomy and physiology. Before attempting to complete any chapter in the *Study and Review Guide,* thoroughly read the corresponding chapter in the textbook, learn the key terms listed at the beginning of each textbook chapter and study your lecture notes. You will then be prepared to complete the questions and exercises that are provided for each chapter.

Each chapter in the *Study and Review Guide* begins with a brief overview of the chapter concepts. A variety of questions is offered to help you cover the material effectively. These questions include multiple choice, true-false, matching, short answer, clinical challenges, labeling, and crossword puzzles.

Multiple Choice

For each multiple choice question, there is only one correct answer out of the choices given. Circle the correct choice.

True or False

Read each statement carefully and write true or false in the blank provided

Matching

Match each numbered term or statement in the left-hand column with its corresponding lettered term or statement in the right-hand column. Write the correct letters in the blanks provided.

Fill in the Blanks

Fill-in-the-blank questions ask you to recall missing word(s) and insert it (them) into the answer blank(s) These questions may involve sentences or paragraphs.

Identify the Term that Does Not Belong

In questions that ask you to identify the incorrect term, three words are given that relate to each other in structure and function, and one more word is included that has no relationship to the other three terms. You are asked to circle the term that does not relate to the others. An example might be: iris, stapes, cornea, and retina. You would circle stapes because all other terms refer to the eye.

Application Questions

Application questions ask you to make a judgment based on the information in the chapter. These questions may ask you how you would respond to a situation or to suggest a possible diagnosis for a set of symptoms.

Labeling Exercises

Labeling exercises present diagrams with parts that are not identified. According to the directions given, fill in the appropriate labels on the numbered lines or match the numbers with the lettered list of terms provided.

Crossword Puzzles

Vocabulary words from the Key Terms section in each chapter of the text have been developed into crossword puzzles. This exercise encourages recall and proper spelling.

One Last Quick Check

This section selects questions from throughout the chapter to provide you with a final review of the chapter. This mini-test gives you an overview of your knowledge of the chapter after completing all of the other sections.

Finally, after completing the exercises in a chapter, check your answers. Answers can be found in the back of the book. Each answer is referenced to the appropriate text page. Additionally, questions are grouped into specific topics that correspond to the text. Each major topic of the Study and Review Guide provides references to specific areas of the text, so if you are having difficulty with a particular grouping of questions you have a specific reference area to assist you with remedial work. This allows you to identify your area of weakness accurately. Good luck!

FIGURE ACKNOWLEDGMENTS

Brundage, D.J.: *Renal disorders*, St. Louis, 1992, Mosby.
Unn 28-1
Unn 28-2

Acknowledgments

I wish to express my appreciation to the staff at Elsevier, and especially to Tom Wilhelm, Jeff Downing, and Jennifer Stoces for their guidance and support. My continued admiration and thanks to Gary Thibodeau and Kevin Patton for another outstanding edition of their text. Your time and dedication to science education will, hopefully, help improve the quality of health care for our future and instill in each student a deep appreciation for the wonders of the human body.

My thanks to Brian, whose encouragement keeps me on task, whose discussions keep my creative juices flowing and whose love makes my life special.

My thanks, as well, to Bill Fortner who is always there whenever I need him.

To my mother, my daughter Amanda, and grandchildren Billy and Maddie this book is dedicated with gratitude and love. You are the roots and fruit of my tree of life.

Linda Swisher, RN, EdD

Contents

CHAPTER 1

Organization of the Body

The study of anatomy and physiology involves the structure and function of an organism and the relationship of its parts. It begins with a basic organization of the body into different structural levels. Beginning with the smallest level (the cell) and progressing to the largest, most complex level (the system), this chapter familiarizes you with the terminology and the levels of organization needed to facilitate the study of the body in parts or as a whole.

It is also important to be able to identify and describe specific body areas or regions as we progress in this field. The anatomical position is used as a reference when dissecting the body into planes, regions, or cavities. The terminology defined in this chapter allows you to describe the areas efficiently and accurately.

Finally, the process of homeostasis is reviewed. This state of relative constancy in the chemical composition of body fluids is necessary for good health. In fact, the very survival of the body depends on the successful maintenance of homeostasis.

I—ANATOMY AND PHYSIOLOGY AND CHARACTERISTICS OF LIFE

Multiple Choice—select the best answer.

1. *Anatomy* refers to:
   a. using devices to investigate parameters such as heart rate and blood pressure.
   b. investigating human structure via dissection and other methods.
   c. studying the unusual manner in which an organism responds to painful stimuli.
   d. examining the chemistry of life.

2. *Systemic anatomy* refers to anatomical investigation:
   a. at a microscopic level.
   b. that begins in the head and neck and concludes at the feet.
   c. that approaches the study of the body by systems: groups of organs having a common function.
   d. at the cellular level.

3. *Physiology* refers to the:
   a. nature of human function.
   b. structure of the human form.
   c. evolution of human thought.
   d. accuracy of measuring the human physique.

4. The removal of waste products in the body is achieved by a process known as: ___ and
   a. secretion.
   b. excretion.
   c. circulation.
   d. conductivity.

5. *Metabolism* is the:
   a. exchange of gases in the blood.
   b. formation of new cells in the body to permit growth.
   c. sum total of all physical and chemical reactions occurring in the body.
   d. production and delivery of specialized substances for diverse body functions.

▶ *If you had difficulty with this section, review pages 7-9.*

II—LEVELS OF ORGANIZATION

Multiple Choice—select the best answer.

6. Beginning with the smallest level, the levels of organization of the body are:
   a. cellular, chemical, tissue, organelle, organ, system, organism.
   b. cellular, chemical, organelle, organ, tissue, organism, system.
   c. chemical, cellular, organelle, organ, system, organism.
   d. chemical, organelle, cellular, tissue, organ, system, organism.

7. Molecules are:
   a. combinations of atoms forming larger chemical aggregates.
   b. electrons orbiting a nucleus.
   c. a complex of electrons arranged in orderly shells.
   d. composed of cellular organelles.

8. Mitochondria, Golgi apparatus, and endoplasmic reticulum are examples of:
   a. macromolecules.
   b. cytoplasm.
   c. organelles.
   d. nuclei.

9. Blood production is a function of which system?
   a. circulatory
   b. respiratory
   c. skeletal
   d. urinary

10. Support and movement are functions of which systems?
    a. respiratory, digestive, and urinary systems
    b. reproductive and urinary systems
    c. skeletal and muscular systems
    d. cardiovascular and lymphatic/immune systems

Matching—match the term with the proper selection.

a. many similar cells that act together to perform a common function
b. the most complex units that make up the body
c. a group of several different kinds of tissues arranged to perform a special function
d. collections of molecules that perform a function
e. the smallest "living" units of structure and function

11. _____ organelle

12. __e__ cells

13. __a__ tissue

14. __c__ organ

15. __b__ systems

Matching—match each system with its corresponding functions.

a. support and movement
b. communication, control, and integration
c. reproduction and development
d. transportation and defense
e. respiration, nutrition, and excretion

16. _____   integumentary system

17. _____   skeletal system

18. _____   muscular system

19. _____   nervous system

20. _____   endocrine system

21. _____   digestive system

22. _____   respiratory system

23. _____   cardiovascular system

24. _____   lymphatic system

25. _____   urinary system

26. _____   reproductive system

▷ *If you had difficulty with this section, review pages 9-12.*

III—ANATOMICAL POSITION, BODY CAVITIES, BODY REGIONS, ANATOMICAL TERMS, AND BODY PLANES

Multiple Choice—select the best answer.

27. In the anatomical position the subject is:
    a. seated with the head facing forward.
    b. standing with the arms at the sides and palms facing forward.
    c. seated with arms parallel to the ground.
    d. standing with the arms at the sides and palms facing backward.

28. The dorsal body cavity contains the:
    a. brain and spinal cord.
    b. abdominal organs.
    c. pelvic organs.
    d. thoracic organs.

29. The ventral body cavity contains the:
    a. thoracic and abdominopelvic cavities.
    b. thoracic cavity only.
    c. abdominopelvic cavity only.
    d. brain and spinal cord.

30. The axial portion of the body consists of:
    a. arms, neck, and torso.
    b. neck, torso, and legs.
    c. torso, arms, and legs.
    d. head, neck, and torso.

31. The abdominopelvic cavity contains all of the following *EXCEPT* the:
    a. kidneys.
    b. pancreas.
    c. lungs.
    d. urinary bladder.

32. The mediastinum contains all of the following *EXCEPT* the:
    a. esophagus.
    b. aorta.
    c. lungs.
    d. trachea.

33. Visceral peritoneum would cover which of the following organs?
    a. heart.
    b. liver.
    c. lungs.
    d. brain.

34. A sagittal section would divide the body into:
    a. upper and lower parts.
    b. right and left sides.
    c. front and back portions.
    d. none of the above.

35. A coronal section would divide the body into:
    a. upper and lower parts.
    b. right and left sides.
    c. front and back portions.
    d. none of the above.

36. *Inguinal* is a term referring to which body region?
    a. anterior portion of elbow
    b. armpit
    c. posterior knee
    d. groin

Circle the correct answer.

37. The stomach is (superior or inferior) to the diaphragm.

38. The nose is located on the (anterior or posterior) surface of the body.

39. The lungs lie (medial or lateral) to the heart.

40. The elbow lies (proximal or distal) to the forearm.

41. The skin is (superficial or deep) to the muscles below it.

42. A midsagittal plane divides the body into (equal or unequal) parts.

43. A frontal plane divides the body into (anterior and posterior or superior and inferior) sections.

44. A transverse plane divides the body into (right and left or upper and lower) sections.

45. A coronal plane may also be referred to as a (sagittal or frontal) plane.

Matching—select the correct term from the choices given and insert the letter in the answer blank.

a. ventral cavity   b. dorsal cavity

46. _____ thoracic

47. _____ cranial

48. _____ abdominal

49. _____ pelvic

50. _____ mediastinum

51. _____ pleural

Labeling—using the terms provided, label the anatomical directions on the illustration below.

anterior   posterior   ventral   dorsal
distal   proximal   superior   inferior
lateral   medial   midline   sagittal plane
coronal plane frontal plane transverse plane cross section

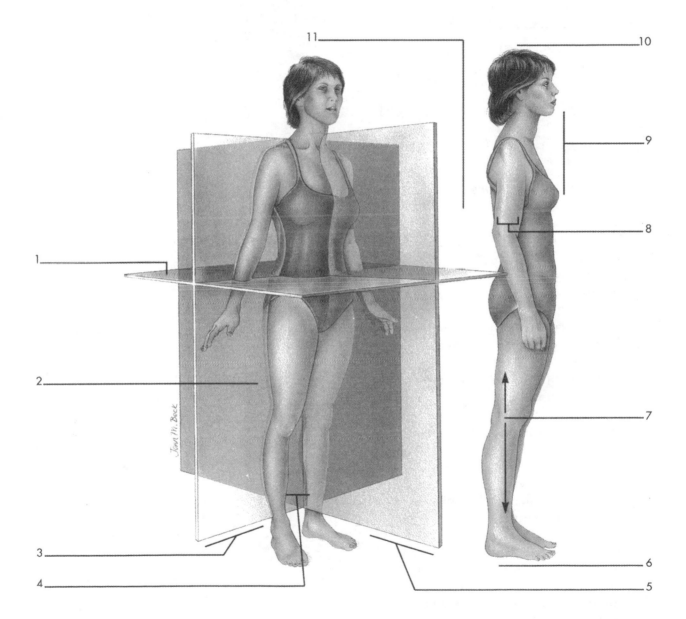

Labeling—label the various body cavities on the diagram below.

▷ *If you had difficulty with this section, review pages 12-18.*

IV—HOMEOSTASIS AND HOMEOSTATIC MECHANISMS OF CONTROL

Multiple Choice—select the best answer.

52. *Homeostasis* can be defined as the:
    a. relatively constant state maintained by the body.
    b. overall contribution of an organ system.
    c. external stimuli that evoke a disruption to an organism.
    d. lack of cytoplasm within a plasma membrane.

53. Which of the following is *NOT* a component of a feedback control loop?
    a. sensory mechanism
    b. integrating, or control center
    c. effector mechanism
    d. stressor stimulator

54. Negative feedback control systems:
    a. oppose a change.
    b. accelerate a change.
    c. ignore a change.
    d. none of the above

55. Positive feedback control systems:
    a. oppose a change.
    b. accelerate a change.
    c. ignore a change.
    d. none of the above.

True or false

56. _____ Any given physiological parameter will never deviate beyond the set point.

57. _____ In the thermostatically regulated furnace example of negative feedback, the furnace functions as the sensor.

58. _____ Negative feedback systems are inhibitory.

59. _____ The process of childbirth, in which the baby's head causes increased stretching of the reproductive tract, which in turn feeds back to the brain, thus triggering the release of oxytocin, is an example of positive feedback.

▷ *If you had difficulty with this section, review pages 20-26.*

ONE LAST QUICK CHECK

Multiple Choice—select the best answer.

79. The body's ability to continuously respond to changes in the environment and maintain consistency in the internal environment is called:
    a. homeostasis.
    b. superficial.
    c. structural levels.
    d. none of the above.

80. The regions frequently used by health professionals to locate pain or tumors divides the abdomen into four basic areas called:
    a. planes.
    b. cavities.
    c. pleural.
    d. quadrants.

81. A lengthwise plane running from front to back that divides the body into right and left sides is called:
    a. transverse.
    b. coronal.
    c. frontal.
    d. sagittal.

82. A study of the functions of living organisms and their parts is called:
    a. physiology.
    b. chemistry.
    c. biology.
    d. none of the above.

83. Which of the following structures does *NOT* lie within the abdominopelvic cavity?
    a. right iliac region
    b. left antecubital region
    c. left lumbar region
    d. hypogastric region

84. The dorsal body cavity contains components of the:
    a. reproductive system.
    b. digestive system.
    c. respiratory system.
    d. nervous system.

85. If your reference point is "nearest the trunk of the body" versus "farthest from the trunk of the body," where does the elbow lie in relation to the wrist?
    a. anterior
    b. posterior
    c. distal
    d. proximal

86. The buttocks are often used as injection sites. This region can also be called:
    a. sacral.
    b. buccal.
    c. cutaneous.
    d. gluteal.

87. Which of the following is *NOT* a component of the axial subdivision of the body?
    a. upper extremity
    b. neck
    c. trunk
    d. head

88. A synonym for medial is:
    a. toward the side.
    b. in front of.
    c. midline.
    d. anterior.

CHAPTER 2

The Chemical Basis of Life

Although anatomy can be studied without knowledge of chemistry, it is hard to imagine an understanding of physiology without a basic comprehension of chemical reactions in the body. Trillions of cells make up the various levels of organization in the body. Our health and survival depend upon the proper chemical maintenance in the cytoplasm of our cells.

Chemists use the terms *elements* or *compounds* to describe all of the substances (matter) in and around us. Distinguishing these two terms is the fact that an element cannot be broken down. A compound, on the other hand, is made up of two or more elements and has the ability to be broken down into the elements that form it.

Organic and inorganic compounds are equally important to us. Without organic compounds such as carbohydrates, proteins, and fats, and inorganic compounds such as water, we could not sustain life.

Because we cannot see many of the chemical reactions that take place daily in our bodies, it is sometimes difficult to comprehend the principles involved in initiating them. Chemicals are responsible for directing virtually all of our bodily functions. It is therefore important to master the fundamental concepts of chemistry.

I—BASIC CHEMISTRY

Multiple Choice—select the best answer.

1. Which of the following is *NOT* one of the major elements present in the human body?
   a. oxygen
   b. carbon
   c. iron
   d. hydrogen

2. Which of the following is *NOT* a subatomic particle?
   a. proton
   b. electron
   c. isotope
   d. neutron

3. The total number of electrons in an atom equals the number of:
   a. neutrons in its nucleus.
   b. electrons in its nucleus.
   c. protons in its nucleus.
   d. ions in its nucleus.

4. An atom can be described as chemically inert if its outermost electron shell contains:
   a. three electrons.
   b. five electrons.
   c. six electrons.
   d. eight electrons.

5. Isotopes are atoms of elements that differ in their number of:
   a. protons.
   b. electrons.
   c. neutrons.
   d. nuclei.

6. Ionic bonds are chemical bonds formed by the:
   a. sharing of electrons between atoms.
   b. donation of protons from one atom to another.
   c. transfer of electrons from one atom to another.
   d. acceptance of protons from one atom to another.

7. Chemical bonds formed by the sharing of electrons are called:
   a. ionic.
   b. covalent.
   c. hydrogen.
   d. electronic.

8. A chemical reaction in which substances combine to form more complex substances is called:
   a. synthesis.
   b. decomposition.
   c. exchange.
   d. reversible.

True or false

9. _____ *Matter* is a term used by chemists to describe all the materials or substances around us.

10. _____ *Atomic weight* refers to the number of protons plus the number of neutrons in an atom.

11. ___F___ Sodium chloride is an example of a covalent bond.

12. _____ Hydrogen bonds form from an equal charge distribution within a molecule.

13. _____ The digestion of food is an example of a decomposition reaction.

Identify the following elements:

14. _____ O

15. _____ Ca

16. _____ K

17. _____ Na

18. _____ Mg

19. _____ Fe

20. _____ Se

▷ *If you had difficulty with this section, review pages 38-45.*

II—METABOLISM

Matching—select the best answer.

a. Breaks down larger food molecules into smaller units
b. The form of energy that cells generally use
c. All the chemical reactions that occur in body cells
d. Joins simple molecules together to form more complex ones
e. Key reaction during anabolism

21. _____ Catabolism

22. _____ Anabolism

23. _____ ATP

24. _____ Metabolism

25. _____ Dehydration synthesis

▷ *If you had difficulty with this section, review pages 45-46.*

III—INORGANIC MOLECULES

Multiple Choice—select the best answer.

26. Water plays a key role in such processes as:
    a. cell permeability.
    b. active transport of materials.
    c. secretion.
    d. all of the above.

27. Which of the following is *NOT* a property of water?
    a. strong polarity
    b. high specific heat
    c. high heat of vaporization
    d. strong acidity

28. Acids:
    a. are proton donors.
    b. dye litmus blue.
    c. release hydrogen ions when in an aqueous solution.
    d. accept electrons when in an aqueous solution.

29. Substances that accept hydrogen ions are referred to as:
    a. acids.
    b. bases.
    c. buffers.
    d. salts.

30. The constancy of the pH homeostatic mechanism is caused by the presence of substances called:
    a. salts.
    b. bases.
    c. buffers.
    d. acids.

True or false

31. ___F___ The pH scale indicates the degree of acidity or alkalinity of a solution.

32. ___T___ Milk is acid on the pH scale.

33. ___T___ Litmus will turn red in the presence of an acid.

34. _____ The basic substance of each cell is water.

35. ___F___ Oxygen and carbon dioxide are examples of organic compounds.

 If you had difficulty with this section, review pages 45-50.

IV—ORGANIC MOLECULES

Multiple Choice—select the best answer.

36. Which of the following is *NOT* a type of carbohydrate?
    a. monosaccharides
    b. disaccharides
    c. megasaccharides
    d. polysaccharides

37. Which of the following is *INCORRECT* in reference to carbohydrates?
    a. They include substances referred to as *sugars.*
    b. They serve critical structural roles in RNA and DNA.
    c. They represent a primary source of chemical energy for body cells.
    d. They are replete with nitrogen atoms.

38. Proteins are composed of ____ commonly occurring amino acids.
    a. 8
    b. 12
    c. 20
    d. 24

39. Amino acids frequently become joined by:
    a. peptide bonds.
    b. phospholipid reactions.
    c. degradation synthesis.
    d. none of the above.

40. Which of the following is *NOT* an example of proteins?
    a. hormones
    b. antibodies
    c. urine
    d. enzymes

41. A structural lipid found in a cell membrane is:
    a. triglyceride.
    b. phospholipid.
    c. steroid.
    d. prostaglandin.

42. Which of the following is the correct example of DNA base pairing?
    a. adenine-cytosine
    b. guanine-adenine
    c. adenine-thymine
    d. guanine-thymine

43. A DNA molecule contains each of the following *EXCEPT:*
    a. sugar.
    b. nitrogenous base.
    c. phosphate.
    d. lipid.

44. DNA differs from RNA in that:
    a. RNA contains ribose instead of deoxyribose.
    b. RNA contains thymine instead of uracil.
    c. RNA contains a double polynucleotide strand.
    d. There is no structural difference between DNA and RNA.

True or false

45. _____ Steroids are poorly distributed throughout the body.

46. _____ High-density lipoprotein (HDL) is also called the "good" cholesterol.

47. _____ Protein compounds have no role in defending the body against harmful agents.

48. _____ The nonessential amino acids can be produced from the other amino acids or from simple organic molecules.

49. _____ Enzymes are proteins that function by the "lock and key" model.

50. _____ Prostaglandins are "tissue hormones."

▷ *If you had difficulty with this section, review pages 51-67.*

Crossword Puzzle

Across
1. Acts as a reservoir for H ions
5. DNA or RNA (two words)
9. Small particle of an element
10. Simple form of matter
12. Amino acid
14. Tastes bitter

Down
2. Dissociates in solution to form ions
3. Releases hydrogen when in solution
4. _____ bond/electrocovalent bond
6. Sugar or starch
7. Chemical catalysts
8. _____ bond/shares electron pairs between atoms
11. Fat
13. Electrically charged atom

APPLYING WHAT YOU KNOW

51. Amanda and Bill own a home that was recently discovered to contain very high levels of radon. Where in the house would these levels be greatest? What could be done to eliminate the radon? What is the family at greatest risk for?

52. Kim just finished preparing a meal of pan-fried hamburgers for her family. While the frying pan was still hot, she poured the liquid grease into a metal container to cool. Later she noticed that the liquid oil had solidified as it cooled. Explain the chemistry of why the now room-temperature fat was solid.

DID YOU KNOW?

• After a vigorous workout, your triglycerides fall 10–20% and your HDL increases by the same percentage for 2–3 hours.

ONE LAST QUICK CHECK

Matching—identify each term with its corresponding description or definition.

a. atomic number
b. base pairs
c. electrolyte
d. high-energy bonds
e. isotopes
f. nucleotide
g. octet rule
h. polarity
i. polymers

53. _____ Atoms of the same element but with different atomic weights (because their nuclei contain different numbers of neutrons).

54. _____ Adenine-thymine and guanine-cytosine are examples of _____ present in DNA.

55. _____ Atoms with fewer than eight electrons in their valence shell will attempt to lose, gain, or share electrons with other atoms to achieve stability.

56. _____ The number of protons in an atom's nucleus.

57. _____ Any large molecule made up of many identical small molecules.

58. _____ Components of DNA and RNA that are composed of sugar, a nitrogenous base, and a phosphate group.

59. _____ Chemical property that allows water to act as an effective solvent.

60. _____ Large group of inorganic compounds including acids, bases, and salts.

Matching—select the best answer.

a. protein
b. carbohydrate
c. lipid

61. _____ ribose
62. _____ steroids
63. _____ amino acid
64. _____ glycerol
65. _____ monosaccharides
66. _____ phospholipids
67. _____ enzymes

Matching—select the best answer.

a. acid   b. base

68. _____ litmus turns blue
69. _____ "proton donor"
70. _____ bitter taste
71. _____ "proton acceptor"
72. _____ releases a hydrogen ion

Labeling—label the following microscope diagram using the terms provided.

fine focus   coarse focus   mechanical stage
light source   objective lens   condensor lens
specimen on slide   ocular lens

Labeling—from memory, label the parts of the typical cell on the diagram below.

▷ *If you had difficulty with this section, review pages 82-96.*

II—CYTOSKELETON

Fill in the blanks.

21. _____ is the cell's internal supporting framework.

22. _____ are the smallest cell fibers.

23. The thickest of the cell fibers are tiny, hollow tubes called _____.

24. The _____ is an area of the cytoplasm near the nucleus that coordinates the building and breaking of microtubules in the cell.

25. _____, _____, and _____ are cell extensions that appear on certain types of cells.

26. When membrane channels of adjacent plasma membranes adhere to others, the formation is known as _____ _____.

27. _____ hold skin together.

▷ *If you had difficulty with this section, review pages 93-97.*

Crossword Puzzle

Across

2. _____ apparatus/synthesizes carbohydrates
4. Power plants
5. Gel-like substance within the cell
7. Contains DNA
8. Area of cytoplasm near the nucleus
9. Rough and smooth (abbrev.)

Down

1. Protein factory
3. _____ membrane/surrounds the cell
6. Cell's digestive system

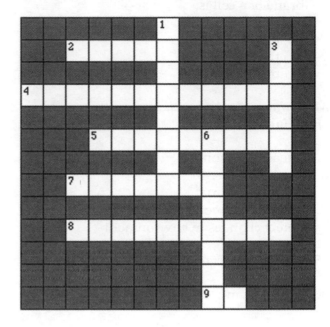

APPLYING WHAT YOU KNOW

28. Brian is a sedentary, overweight cigarette smoker who has chest pain whenever he exerts himself. Upon examination, his cardiologist determines that Brian is suffering from heart disease. Which receptors in the cells that line the blood vessels of his heart are responsible? What type of cholesterol is responsible?

    What other diseases may he be at risk for?

29. After several weeks of exercising in the weight room, Valerie notices that she has not only become stronger, but quite muscular as well. Which organelle has increased its density in the cytoplasm of her muscles in response to a greater demand for ATP production?

    a) ribosome
    b) nucleolus
    c) mitochondria
    d) lysosome

DID YOU KNOW

- The largest single cell in the human body is the female sex cell, the ovum. The smallest single cell in the human body is the male sex cell, the sperm.

ONE LAST QUICK CHECK

Multiple Choice—select the best answer.

30. Which of the following cellular extensions is required when absorption is important?
    a. cilia
    b. microvilli
    c. flagella
    d. none of the above

31. Movement of the ovum within the female reproductive tract is largely as a result of:
    a. the flagella extending from the ovum.
    b. the cilia extending from the ovum.
    c. the cilia lining the uterine tubes.
    d. none of the above.

32. Skin cells are held tightly together by:
    a. gap junctions.
    b. desmosomes.
    c. tight junctions.
    d. adhesions.

33. Ribosomes are attached to:
    a. lysosomes.
    b. rough endoplasmic reticulum.
    c. peroxisomes.
    d. cilia.

34. The phospholipid area of the plasma membrane of a cell is:
    a. single-layered.
    b. bilayered.
    c. trilayered.
    d. multilayered.

Matching—identify each term with its corresponding definition.

a. release hormones
b. transport oxygen
c. destroy bacteria
d. contract for movement
e. detect changes in environment

35. _____   nerve cells

36. _____   muscle cells

37. _____   red blood cells

38. _____   gland cells

39. _____   immune cells

Fill in the blanks.

40. A typical or _____
    cell exhibits the most important characteristics of cell types.

41. _____ is the
    term used to describe "water loving."

42. _____ is the
    process that allows a message to be carried
    across a membrane.

43. _____ detoxify harmful substances that enter cells.

44. The _____ is
    one of the largest cell structures and occupies the central portion of the cell.

CHAPTER 4

Physiology of Cells

Cells, just like humans, require water, food, gases, elimination of wastes, and numerous other substances and processes in order to survive. Cells must transport the substances within the cytoplasm and across cell membranes. The movement of these substances in and out of the cell is accomplished by two primary methods: passive transport and active transport. In passive transport, no cellular energy is required to effect movement through the cell membrane. However, in active transport, cellular energy is necessary to provide movement through the cell membrane.

Cell reproduction completes the study of cells. A basic explanation of DNA, the "hereditary molecule," gives us a proper respect for the capability of the cell to transmit physical and mental traits from generation to generation. Reproduction of the cell—mitosis—is a complex process requiring several stages. These stages are outlined and diagrammed in the text to facilitate learning. An understanding of cell physiology will assist you in your comprehension of the physiology of the body as a whole.

I—MOVEMENT OF SUBSTANCES THROUGH CELL MEMBRANES

Multiple Choice—select the best answer.

1. Which of the following is *NOT* a passive transport process?
   a. dialysis
   b. osmosis
   c. filtration
   d. pinocytosis

2. Diffusion of water through a selectively permeable membrane in the presence of at least one impermeant solute is referred to as:
   a. diffusion.
   b. osmosis.
   c. phagocytosis.
   d. dialysis.

3. The trapping of bacteria by specialized white blood cells is an example of:
   a. pinocytosis.
   b. exocytosis.
   c. phagocytosis.
   d. none of the above.

4. A hypertonic solution is one that contains:
   a. a greater concentration of solute than the cell.
   b. the same concentration of solute as the cell.
   c. a lesser concentration of solute as the cell.
   d. none of the above.

5. The force of a fluid pushing against a surface could be described as:
   a. facilitated diffusion.
   b. hydrostatic pressure.
   c. hypostatic pressure.
   d. none of the above.

True or false

6. _____ Facilitated diffusion is a metabolically expensive process.

7. _____ The sodium-potassium pump is an example of an active transport process.

8. _____ Cellular secretion can be achieved by exocytosis.

9. _____ Solutes are particles dissolved in a solvent.

10. _____ Osmosis is a form of filtration that results in the separation of small and large solute particles.

Matching—identify each item with its corresponding description.

a. isotonic
b. hypertonic
c. hypotonic
d. diffusion
e. endocytosis

11. _____ solution that draws water from a cell

12. _____ two fluids that have the same potential osmotic pressure

13. _____ solution that causes cells to swell

14. _____ passive transport

15. _____ active transport

Labeling—match each term with its corresponding number in the following diagram of cellular respiration.

____ aerobic

____ glucose

____ mitochondrion

____ anaerobic

____ pyruvic acid

____ citric acid cycle

____ lactic acid

____ O$_2$

____ ATP

____ transition

____ H$_2$O

____ acetyl CoA

▷ *If you had difficulty with this section, review pages 103-112.*

II—CELL METABOLISM

Multiple Choice—select the best answer.

16. Enzymes that cause essential chemical reactions to occur are called:
    a. metabolic agents.
    b. catalysts.
    c. substrates.
    d. initiators.

17. In the DNA molecule, a sequence of three base pairs forms a(n):
    a. codon.
    b. anticodon.
    c. polymerase.
    d. none of the above.

18. Transcription can be best described as the:
    a. synthesis of tRNA.
    b. reading of mRNA codons by tRNA.
    c. synthesis of mRNA.
    d. synthesis of polypeptides at a ribosomal site.

19. Which of the following statements is true?
    a. Complex polypeptide chains form tRNA.
    b. The site of transcription is within the nucleus, whereas the site of translation is in the cytoplasm.
    c. Uracil is present in DNA in the place of thymine.
    d. None of the above is true.

20. A DNA molecule is characterized by all of the following *EXCEPT*:
    a. double-helix shape.
    b. obligatory base pairing.
    c. ribose sugar.
    d. phosphate groups.

21. Which of the following is *NOT* a characteristic of RNA?
    a. It is single-stranded.
    b. It contains uracil and not thymine.
    c. The obligatory base pairs are adenine-uracil and guanine-cytosine.
    d. Its molecules are larger than those of DNA.

True or false

22. _____ The three processes that comprise cellular respiration are glycolysis, the citric acid cycle, and the electron transport system.

23. _____ The portion of an enzyme molecule that chemically "fits" the substrate molecule(s) is referred to as the *active site*.

24. _____ One significant similarity between RNA and DNA is that they both are shaped as a double helix.

25. _____ The "lock and key" model is used to describe how DNA base pairs align.

26. _____ Protein anabolism is a major cellular activity.

27. _____ The citric acid cycle is also known as the *Krebs cycle*.

28. _____ Glycolysis is aerobic.

Matching—identify the term related to protein synthesis with its corresponding definition.

a. mRNA
b. ribosome
c. tRNA
d. translation
e. transcription
f. complimentary base pair

29. _____ process that occurs when the double strands of a DNA segment separate and RNA nucleotides pair with the DNA nucleotides

30. _____ the type of RNA that carries information in groups of three nucleotides called codons, each of which codes for a specific amino acid

31. _____ the type of RNA that has an anticodon and binds to a base pair–specific amino acid

32. _____ the process involving the movement of mRNA with respect to the ribosome

33. _____ uracil-adenine

34. _____ the site of translation

Labeling—label the following DNA molecule.

▷ *If you had difficulty with this section, review pages 114-125.*

III—GROWTH AND REPRODUCTION OF CELLS

Multiple Choice—select the best answer.

35. Nucleic acids are synthesized directly on the DNA molecule with the help of:
    a. enzymes.
    b. prophase.
    c. neoplasms.
    d. lipids.

36. The correct order of mitosis is:
    a. prophase, metaphase, anaphase, telophase.
    b. anaphase, telophase, metaphase, prophase.
    c. prophase, anaphase, metaphase, telophase.
    d. none of the above.

37. The total of 46 chromosomes per cell is referred to as:
    a. haploid.
    b. diploid.
    c. myoid.
    d. none of the above.

38. Which of the following terms is synonymous with *tumor*?
    a. anaplasia
    b. hyperplasia
    c. neoplasm
    d. benign

True or false

39. _____ *Gamete* is a term referring to the point of attachment of newly replicated DNA molecules.

40. _____ Normal mitosis results in daughter cells that are genetically identical to the parent cell.

41. _____ It is during meiosis II that the number of chromosomes is halved.

42. _____ Telophase is the "completion phase" of mitosis.

43. _____ *Hyperplasia* refers to an increase in cell size, whereas *hypertrophy* refers to an increase in cell number.

▶ *If you had difficulty with this section, review pages 130-136.*

IV—MECHANISMS OF DISEASE

True or false

44. _____ Diabetes mellitus is a disorder of cell membrane receptors.

45. _____ Genetic disorders are mutations in a cell's genetic code.

46. _____ Cystic fibrosis is a condition in which chloride ion pumps in the plasma membrane are missing.

47. _____ Viruses do not contain DNA or RNA.

48. _____ A blood disease caused by the production of abnormal hemoglobin is known as *sickle cell anemia*.

Labeling—on the following diagram, label the phases of mitosis. Remember that interphase and DNA replication occur before mitosis begins!

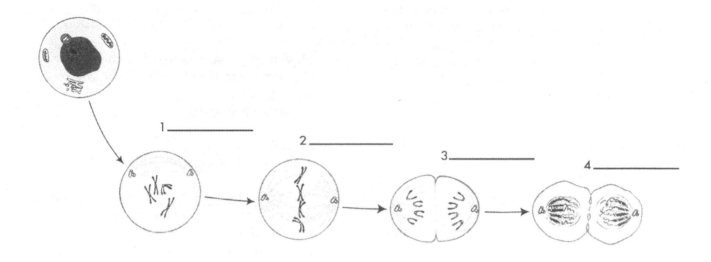

1 _____

2 _____

3 _____

4 _____

▷ *If you had difficulty with this section, review pages 138-139.*

Crossword Puzzle

Across
1. Sum of chemical reactions in a cell
4. Concentration _____ measures difference from one area to another
7. Cell reproduction
8. Passive process
9. "Traps" extracellular material and brings it into cell

Down
2. Movement that requires cell energy (two words)
3. Diffusion of water
5. Chemical catalyst
6. Sex cell reproduction

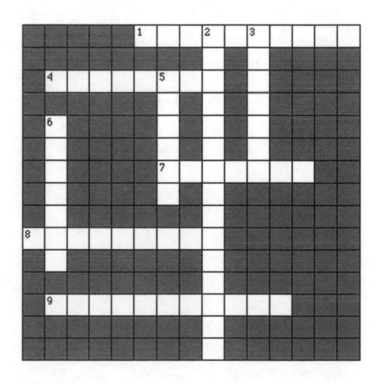

APPLYING WHAT YOU KNOW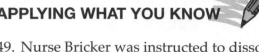

49. Nurse Bricker was instructed to dissolve a pill in a small amount of liquid medication. As she dropped the capsule into the liquid, she was interrupted by the telephone. On her return to the medication cart, she found the medication completely dissolved and apparently scattered evenly throughout the liquid.

    This phenomenon did not surprise her because she was aware from her knowledge of cell transport that _____ had created this distribution.

50. Bobbi ran in the Boston marathon. During the race she lost a lot of fluids through perspiration and became dehydrated. Would you expect her cells to shrink, swell, or remain the same?

DID YOU KNOW ?

- A human can detect one drop of perfume diffused throughout a three-room apartment.

ONE LAST QUICK CHECK ✔

Multiple Choice—select the best answer.

51. In which stage of mitosis do chromosomes move to opposite ends of the cells along the spindle fibers?
    a. anaphase
    b. metaphase
    c. prophase
    d. telophase

52. The synthesis of proteins by ribosomes using information coded in the mRNA molecule is called:
    a. translation.
    b. transcription.
    c. replication.
    d. crenation.

53. The energy required for active transport processes is obtained from:
    a. ATP.
    b. DNA.
    c. diffusion.
    d. osmosis.

54. Movement of substances from a region of high concentration to a region of low concentration is:
    a. active transport.
    b. passive transport.
    c. cellular energy.
    d. concentration gradient.

55. Osmosis is the _____ of water across a selectively permeable membrane.
    a. filtration
    b. equilibrium
    c. active transport
    d. diffusion

56. A molecule or other agent that alters enzyme function by changing its shape is called:
    a. an allosteric effector.
    b. kinases.
    c. an anabolic agent.
    d. a proenzyme.

57. Glycolysis is a catabolic pathway that begins with glucose and ends with:
    a. oxygen.
    b. filtration
    c. pyruvic acid.
    d. sodium.

58. Which movement always occurs down a hydrostatic pressure gradient?
    a. osmosis
    b. filtration
    c. dialysis
    d. facilitated diffusion

59. The uphill movement of a substance through a living cell membrane is:
    a. osmosis.
    b. diffusion.
    c. active transport.
    d. passive transport.

60. The ion pump is an example of which type of movement?
    a. gravity
    b. hydrostatic pressure
    c. active transport
    d. passive transport

61. An example of a cell that uses phagocytosis is the:
    a. white blood cell.
    b. red blood cell.
    c. muscle cell
    d. bone cell.

62. A saline solution that contains a higher concentration of salt than living red blood cells would be:
    a. hypotonic.
    b. hypertonic.
    c. isotonic.
    d. homeostatic.

63. A red blood cell becomes engorged with water and will eventually lyse, releasing hemoglobin into the solution. This solution is _____ to the red blood cell.
    a. hypotonic
    b. hypertonic
    c. isotonic
    d. homeostatic

Circle the word or phrase that does not belong.

64. DNA   adenine   uracil   thymine

65. RNA   ribose   thymine   uracil

66. translation   protein synthesis mRNA   interphase

67. cleavage furrow   anaphase   prophase   2 daughter cells

68. metaphase   prophase   telophase   gene

CHAPTER 5

Tissues

After successfully completing the study of the cell, you are ready to progress to the next level of anatomical structure: tissues. Four principal types of tissue—epithelial, connective, muscle, and nervous—perform multiple functions to assure that homeostasis is maintained. Among these functions are protection, absorption, excretion, support, insulation, conduction of impulses, movement of bones, and destruction of bacteria. This variety of functions gives us a real appreciation for the complexity of this level.

A macroscopic view confirms this statement as we marvel at the fact that soft, sticky, liquid blood and sturdy compact bone are both considered tissues. Our study continues with the discussion of body membranes and their function for the body. Membranes are thin layers of epithelial and/or connective tissue that cover and protect the body surfaces, line body cavities, and cover the internal surfaces of hollow organs. These major membranes—cutaneous, serous, mucous, and synovial—are also critical to homeostasis and body survival. An understanding of tissues and membranes is necessary to successfully bridge your knowledge between the cell and the study of body organs.

I—PRINCIPAL TYPES OF TISSUES

Multiple Choice—select the best answer.

1. A tissue is:
    a. a membrane that lines body cavities.
    b. a group of similar cells that perform a common function.
    c. a thin sheet of cells embedded in a matrix.
    d. the most complex organizational unit of the body.

2. The four principal types of tissues include all of the following *EXCEPT:*
    a. nervous.
    b. muscle.
    c. cartilage.
    d. connective.

3. The most complex tissue in the body is:
    a. muscle.
    b. blood.
    c. connective.
    d. nervous.

4. The nonliving intercellular material that surrounds tissues is called:
   a. intercellular material.
   b. extracellular matrix.
   c. lacunae.
   d. none of the above.

5. The hollow ball of cells that forms after fertilization is referred to as:
   a. primary germ layer.
   b. blastocyst.
   c. gastrulation.
   d. none of the above.

6. Which tissue lines body cavities and protects body surfaces?
   a. epithelial
   b. connective
   c. muscular
   d. nervous

True or false

7. _____   The biology of tissues is referred to as *histology.*

8. _____   The process by which blastocyst cells move and then differentiate into three primary germ layers is called *gastrulation.*

9. _____   Sweat and sebaceous glands are formed by connective tissue.

10. _____   The three primary germ layers are endoderm, ectoderm, and mesoderm.

▷ *If you had difficulty with this section, review pages 145-147.*

II—EPITHELIAL TISSUE

Multiple Choice—select the best answer.

11. Which of the following is *NOT* a function of membranous epithelium?
    a. secretion
    b. protection
    c. absorption
    d. all are functions of the membranous epithelium

12. Which of the following is *NOT* a structural example of epithelium?
    a. stratified squamous
    b. simple transitional
    c. stratified columnar
    d. pseudostratified columnar

13. The simple columnar epithelium lining the intestines contains plasma membranes that extend into thousands of microscopic extensions called:
    a. villi.
    b. microvilli.
    c. cilia.
    d. flagella.

14. Epithelial cells can be classified according to shape. Which of the following is *NOT* a characteristic shape of epithelium?
    a. cuboidal
    b. rectangular
    c. squamous
    d. columnar

15. Keratinized stratified squamous epithelium is found in the:
    a. mouth.
    b. vagina.
    c. skin.
    d. all of the above.

16. Endocrine glands discharge their products into:
    a. body cavities.
    b. blood.
    c. organ surfaces.
    d. none of the above.

17. Which of the following is *NOT* a functional classification of exocrine glands?
    a. alveolar
    b. apocrine
    c. holocrine
    d. merocrine

18. The functional classification of salivary glands is:
    a. endocrine.
    b. apocrine.
    c. holocrine.
    d. merocrine.

19. This epithelial tissue readily allows diffusion, as in the linings of blood and lymphatic vessels.
    a. simple squamous
    b. stratified squamous
    c. simple columnar
    d. pseudostratified columnar

True or false

20. _____ Epithelial tissue is attached to an underlying layer of connective tissue called the *basement membrane.*

21. _____ Epithelium is rich with blood supply.

22. _____ Exocrine glands discharge their products directly into the blood.

Matching—identify the arrangement of epithelial cells with its corresponding description.

a. simple squamous
b. simple cuboidal
c. simple columnar
d. pseudostratified columnar
e. stratified squamous
f. stratified cuboidal
g. stratified columnar
h. transitional

23. _____ single layer of cube-shaped cells

24. _____ multiple layers of cells with flat cells at the outer surface

25. _____ single layer of cells in which some are tall and thin and able to reach the free surface and others are not

26. _____ layers of cells that appear cube-like when an organ is relaxed and flat or distended by fluid

27. _____ single layer of flat, scalelike cells

28. _____ single layer of tall, thin cells

Labeling—label the following images and identify the principal tissue type of each. Be as specific as possible. Consult your textbook if you need assistance.

Tissue type: _____

1

2

Tissue type: _____

1

2

4

3

5

Tissue type: _____

1

2

3

4

Tissue type: _____

If you had difficulty with this section, review pages 150-159.

III—CONNECTIVE TISSUE

Multiple Choice—select the best answer.

29. Which of the following is *NOT* an example of connective tissue?
    a. transitional
    b. reticular
    c. blood
    d. bone

30. Which of the following fibers is *NOT* found in connective tissue matrix?
    a. collagenous
    b. elastic
    c. fibroblastic
    d. reticular

31. Fibroblasts are usually present in the greatest numbers in which type of tissue?
    a. adipose
    b. areolar
    c. reticular
    d. dense

32. Adipose tissue performs which of the following functions?
    a. insulation
    b. protection
    c. support
    d. all of the above

33. Which of the following connective tissue types forms the framework of the spleen, lymph nodes, and bone marrow?
    a. loose
    b. adipose
    c. reticular
    d. areolar

34. The mature cells of bone are called:
    a. fibroblasts.
    b. osteoclasts.
    c. osteoblasts.
    d. osteocytes.

35. The basic structural unit of bone is the microscopic:
    a. osteon.
    b. lacunae.
    c. lamellae.
    d. canaliculi.

36. Mature bone grows and is reshaped by the simultaneous activity of which two cells?
    a. osteoblasts and osteocytes
    b. osteoblasts and osteoclasts
    c. osteocytes and osteoclasts
    d. none of the above

37. The most prevalent type of cartilage is:
    a. hyaline cartilage.
    b. fibrous cartilage.
    c. elastic cartilage.
    d. none of the above.

38. Which of the following is *NOT* released by injured tissues?
    a. histamine
    b. serotonin
    c. kinins
    d. all of the above are released

True or false

39. _____ The most prevalent types of cells in areolar connective tissue are fibroblasts and macrophages.

40. _____ The terms *osteon* and *Haversian system* are synonymous.

41. _____ The long bones of the body are formed through the process of intramembranous ossification.

42. _____ Cartilage is perhaps the most vascular tissue in the human body.

43. _____ Many researchers believe that one of the most basic factors in the aging process is the change in the molecular structure of collagen.

44. _____ The greater a person's weight while immersed, the higher the body-fat percentage.

Labeling—label the following images and identify the principal tissue type of each. Be as specific as possible. Consult your textbook if you need assistance.

Tissue type: _____

Tissue type: _____

Tissue type: _____

Tissue type: _____

Tissue type: _____

▷ *If you had difficulty with this section, review pages 160-172.*

IV—MUSCLE TISSUE

Matching—identify the type of muscle tissue with its corresponding definition.

a. cardiac muscle
b. skeletal muscle
c. smooth muscle

45. _____ cylindrical, striated, voluntary cells

46. _____ nonstriated, involuntary, narrow fibers with only one nucleus per fiber

47. _____ striated, branching, involuntary cells with intercalated disks

48. _____ responsible for willed body movements

49. _____ also called *visceral muscle*

50. _____ found in the walls of hollow internal organs

Labeling—label the following images and identify the principal tissue type of each. Be as specific as possible. Consult your textbook if you need assistance.

Tissue type: _____

Tissue type: _____

▷ *If you had difficulty with this section, review pages 175-177.*

V—NERVOUS TISSUE

Matching—identify each term with its corresponding description.

a. neuron
b. neuroglia
c. axon
d. soma
e. dendrite

51. _____ the cell body of the neuron

52. _____ supportive cells

53. _____ cell process that transmits nerve impulses away from the cell body

54. _____ the conducting cells of the nervous system

55. _____ cell process that carries nerve impulses toward the cell body

Labeling—label the following image and identify the principal tissue type. Be as specific as possible. Consult your textbook if you need assistance.

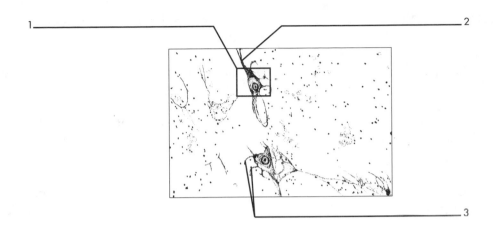

Tissue type: _____

▷ *If you had difficulty with this section, review page 177.*

VI—TISSUE REPAIR

Matching—identify each term with its corresponding description.

a. calor
b. regeneration
c. edema
d. rubor
e. histamine
f. dolor
g. keloid
h. phagocytosis
i. leukocytosis
j. chemotaxis

56. _____   process by which white blood cells engulf and destroy bacteria

57. _____   redness indicating increased blood flow and pooling of blood following injury

58. _____   growth of new tissue (as opposed to scarring)

59. _____   heat resulting from the increased blood flow to the area of injury

60. _____   attraction of leukocytes

61. _____   pain

62. _____   chemical causing increased blood vessel permeability

63. _____   an unusually thick scar

64. _____   increased number of white blood cells

65. _____   the presence of abnormally large amounts of fluid in intercellular tissue spaces

▷ *If you had difficulty with this section, review pages 167 and 178.*

VII—BODY MEMBRANES

Multiple Choice—select the best answer.

66. Which of the following is *NOT* an example of epithelial membrane?
    a. synovial membrane
    b. cutaneous membrane
    c. serous membrane
    d. mucous membrane

67. Pleurisy is a condition that affects which membrane?
    a. cutaneous membrane
    b. serous membrane
    c. mucous membrane
    d. none of the above

True or false

68. _____ Parietal membranes cover the surface of organs.

69. _____ Synovial membrane and bursae are examples of connective tissue membrane.

▷ *If you had difficulty with this section, review pages 179-181.*

VIII—TUMORS AND CANCER

Circle the correct answer.

70. Benign tumors usually grow (slowly or quickly).

71. Malignant tumors (are or are not) encapsulated.

72. An example of a benign tumor that arises from epithelial tissue is (papilloma or lipoma).

73. Malignant tumors that arise from connective tissues are generally called (melanoma or sarcoma).

74. A cancer specialist is an (osteologist or oncologist).

75. Chemotherapy uses (cytotoxic or cachexic) compounds to destroy malignant cells.

▷ *If you had difficulty with this section, review pages 183-185.*

Crossword Puzzle

Across
6. Response to a tissue irritant
8. Provides strength for connective tissue
9. Tissue that contains neurons and neuroglia
10. Membrane that lines surfaces that lead to the exterior
11. Cells that perform a common function
12. Tissue that includes glandular

Down
1. Exocrine
2. "Scaly"
3. Process of primary germ layer's tissue development
4. Tissue that includes adipose
5. Growth of new tissue
7. Membrane that lines body cavities
10. Nonliving intercellular material

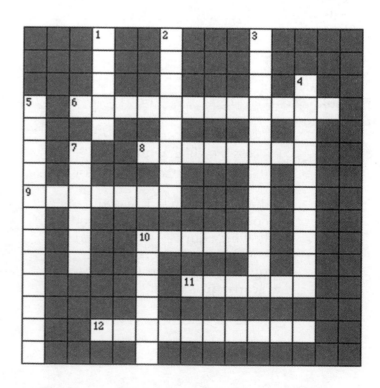

APPLYING WHAT YOU KNOW

76. Holly is a body builder who is obsessed with her physique. She exercises daily and eats a very low-fat diet. A personal fitness trainer has assessed her body fat at 12%. Determine whether she is too lean or too fat. Explain the relationship between her body-fat percentage and lifestyle.

77. Bruce is a sedentary, cigarette smoking, middle-aged man who is complaining of chest pain. Ultimately, he is diagnosed with lung cancer. What tests may have been utilized to determine his diagnosis? Which type of tissues would be involved?

DID YOU KNOW?

- As many as 500,000 Americans die from cancer each year, making it the second leading cause of death in the United States after cardiovascular disease. Half of all cancers are diagnosed in people under the age of 67.

ONE LAST QUICK CHECK ✓

Labeling—label the following images and identify the principal tissue type of each. Be as specific as possible. Consult your textbook if you need assistance.

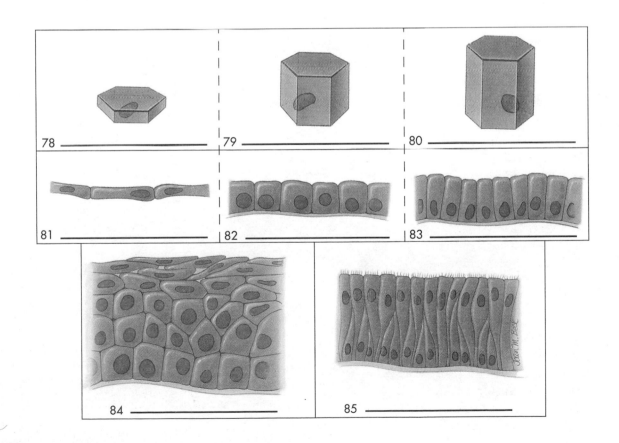

78 _____

79 _____

80 _____

81 _____

82 _____

83 _____

84 _____

85 _____

Multiple Choice—select the best answer.

86. Which of the following is *NOT* an example of connective tissue?
    a. glands
    b. blood
    c. fat
    d. bone

87. Stratified squamous (nonkeratized) epithelium can be found in all of the following *EXCEPT*:
    a. vagina.
    b. mouth.
    c. esophagus.
    d. skin.

88. The most abundant and widespread tissue is:
    a. epithelial.
    b. connective.
    c. muscle.
    d. nervous.

89. Loose connective tissue is also known as:
    a. voluntary.
    b. hyaline.
    c. areolar.
    d. visceral.

90. Tissue that insulates to conserve body heat is:
    a. reticular.
    b. fibrous.
    c. adipose.
    d. osseous.

91. What statement regarding blood is true?
    a. Erythrocytes are white blood cells.
    b. Thrombocytes are also known as *platelets*.
    c. Leukocytes are red blood cells.
    d. Formed elements are known as *plasma*.

92. Cutaneous membrane:
    a. covers body surfaces that are exposed to the external environment.
    b. lines cavities that lead to the outside.
    c. lines closed body cavities.
    d. none of the above.

93. An example of mucous membrane is:
    a. synovial fluid.
    b. bursae.
    c. lining of the respiratory tract.
    d. peritoneum.

CHAPTER 6

Skin and Its Appendages

More of our time, attention, and money are spent on this system than many other. Every time we look into a mirror we become aware of the integumentary system, as we observe our skin, hair, nails, and the appendages that give luster and comfort to this system. The discussion of the skin begins with the structure and function of the two primary layers called the *epidermis* and *dermis*. It continues with an examination of the appendages of the skin, which include the hair, receptors, nails, sebaceous glands, and sudoriferous glands.

Your study of skin concludes with a review of one of the most serious and frequent threats to the skin—burns. An understanding of the integumentary system provides you with an appreciation of the danger that severe burns or trauma can pose to this system.

I—SKIN FUNCTION AND STRUCTURE

Multiple Choice—select the best answer.

1. Beneath the dermis lies a loose layer of skin rich in fat and areolar tissue called the:
   a. dermal-epidermal junction.
   b. hypodermis.
   c. epidermis.
   d. none of the above.

2. The most important cells in the epidermis are the:
   a. keratinocytes.
   b. melanocytes.
   c. Langerhans cells.
   d. dermal papillae.

3. The order of the cells of the epidermis, from superficial to deep, are:
   a. stratum corneum, stratum lucidum, stratum spinosum, stratum granulosum, stratum basale.
   b. stratum corneum, stratum spinosum, stratum lucidum, stratum granulosum, stratum basale.
   c. stratum basale, stratum corneum, stratum lucidum, stratum spinosum, stratum granulosum.
   d. stratum corneum, stratum lucidum, stratum granulosum, stratum spinosum, stratum basale.

4. In which area of the body would you expect to find an especially thick stratum?
   a. back of the hand
   b. thigh
   c. abdomen
   d. sole of the foot

5. In which layer of the skin do cells divide by mitosis to replace cells lost from the outermost surface of the body?
   a. stratum basale
   b. stratum corneum
   c. stratum lucidum
   d. stratum spinosum

6. Smooth muscles that produce "goose pimples" when they contract are:
   a. papillary muscles.
   b. hair muscles.
   c. follicular muscles.
   d. arrector pili muscles.

7. The most common type of skin cancer is:
   a. malignant melanoma.
   b. squamous cell carcinoma.
   c. basal cell carcinoma.
   d. Kaposi sarcoma.

8. Meissner's corpuscles are specialized nerve endings that make it possible for skin to detect:
   a. heat.
   b. cold.
   c. light touch.
   d. deep pressure.

9. The basic determinant of skin color is the quantity of:
   a. keratin.
   b. melanin.
   c. albinin.
   d. none of the above.

10. Which of the following is *NOT* a contributing factor to skin color?
    a. exposure to sunlight
    b. genetics
    c. place of birth
    d. volume of blood in skin capillaries

True or false

11. _____ Most of the body is covered by thick skin.

12. _____ A surgeon would most likely prefer to make an incision parallel to Langer cleavage lines.

13. _____ If the enzyme tyrosinase is absent from birth because of a congenital defect, a condition called *albinism* results.

14. _____ Both benign moles and malignant melanomas are outlined by a distinct border.

15. _____ *Subcutaneous layer* and *hypodermis* are synonymous terms.

Labeling—match each term with its corresponding label on the following diagram of a cross-section of skin.

_____ Meissner's corpuscle   _____ hypodermis

_____ stratum granulosum   _____ opening of sweat ducts

_____ epidermis   _____ dermal papilla

_____ hair shaft   _____ stratum corneum

_____ sebaceous (oil) gland   _____ dermis

_____ stratum basale   _____ hair follicle

▷ *If you had difficulty with this section, review pages 195-204 and 217.*

II—FUNCTIONS OF THE SKIN

Multiple Choice—select the best answer.

16. Which of the following is *NOT* a function of the skin?
    a. sensation
    b. excretion
    c. immunity
    d. all of the above are skin functions

17. Which of the following vitamins is synthesized by the skin?
    a. vitamin A
    b. vitamin B
    c. vitamin C
    d. vitamin D

18. Which of the following is *NOT* a mechanism of heat loss by the skin?
    a. evaporation
    b. radiation
    c. vasoconstriction
    d. convection

19. Langerhans cells are the mechanism of action of which function of skin?
    a. immunity
    b. endocrine
    c. excretion
    d. sensation

20. Which structure compares actual body temperature with set point temperature and then sends out appropriate correction signals to effectors?
    a. pituitary
    b. hypothalamus
    c. thalamus
    d. none of the above

True or false

21. _____ Skin is a minor factor in the body's thermoregulatory mechanism.

22. _____ Skin plays a major role in the overall excretion of body wastes.

23. _____ To help dissipate heat during exercise, sweat production can reach as much as 3 liters per hour.

▷ *If you had difficulty with this section, review pages 208-210.*

III—APPENDAGES OF THE SKIN

Multiple Choice—select the best answer.

24. The developing fetus is covered by an extremely fine, soft hair coat called:
    a. vellus.
    b. lanugo.
    c. fatalis follicle.
    d. none of the above.

25. Which of the following is associated with hair?
    a. sebaceous glands
    b. ceruminous glands
    c. eccrine glands
    d. none of the above

26. Ceruminous glands are found in the:
    a. axillae.
    b. soles of feet.
    c. ear canal.
    d. none of the above.

27. The most numerous, important, and widespread sweat glands in the body are:
    a. apocrine.
    b. eccrine.
    c. ceruminous.
    d. sebaceous.

28. Hair growth is stimulated by:
    a. cutting it frequently.
    b. shaving.
    c. increasing melanin production.
    d. none of the above.

True or false

29. _____ The hair follicle is an extension of the epidermis into the dermis, forming a small tube.

30. _____ The inner core of the hair is called the *cortex.*

31. _____ Sweat, or sudoriferous, glands are the most numerous of the skin glands.

32. _____ One of the factors associated with male pattern baldness is testosterone.

33. _____   Growth of nails is due to mitosis in the stratum germinativum.

▷ *If you had difficulty with this section, review pages 210-215.*

IV—SKIN DISORDERS

Matching—identify the term with the corresponding description.

a. papilloma
b. furuncle
c. ringworm
d. hard skin
e. symptom of underlying condition
f. staph or strep infection
g. bedsores
h. hives

34. _____   impetigo

35. _____   tinea

36. _____   warts

37. _____   boils

38. _____   decubitus ulcers

39. _____   urticaria

40. _____   scleroderma

41. _____   eczema

Fill in the blanks.

42. _____ is the term associated with an unusually high body temperature.

43. _____ _____ occurs when the body loses a large amount of fluid resulting from heat-loss mechanisms.

44. _____ _____ is also known as *sunstroke.*

45. Local damage caused by extremely low temperatures is referred to as _____.

▷ *If you had difficulty with this section, review pages 216-222.*

IV—BURNS

Multiple Choice—select the best answer.

46. The "rule of palms" assumes that the palm size of a burn victim equals about ____ of total body surface area.
    a. 1%
    b. 2%
    c. 5%
    d. none of the above

47. Blisters, severe pain, and generalized swelling are characteristic of which type of burn?
    a. first-degree burns
    b. second-degree burns
    c. third-degree burns
    d. none of the above

True or false

48. _____   According to the "rule of nines," the body is divided into nine areas of 9%.

49. _____   Immediately after injury, third-degree burns hurt less than second-degree burns.

Matching—identify each term with its corresponding description.

A 1st° burn is described ny which of the follow up? al is also called a full-thickness burn.

a. first-degree burn
b. second-degree burn
c. third-degree burn
d. partial-thickness burn
e. full-thickness burn

50. _C_   destroys both epidermis and dermis and may involve underlying tissue

51. _A_   involves only the epidermis

52. _D_   another name for first- and second-degree burns

53. _B_   damage to epidermis and upper layers of dermis with blisters

54. _E_   Another name for third-degree burn

Labeling—using the "rule of nines" method, label the following diagram to estimate the amount of skin surface for each area.

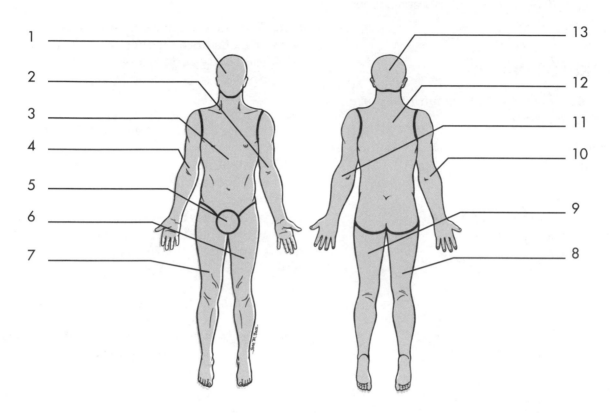

▷ *If you had difficulty with this section, review pages 221-223.*

Crossword Puzzle

Across
6. Tube that contains the hair root (two words)
8. Skin
11. Outer layer of skin
12. "Layer"

Down
1. Layer beneath the dermis
2. Appendage of skin
3. Determines skin color
4. Sudoriferous gland (two words)
5. Water-repellent protein
7. Gland that secretes oil
9. Keratinized epithelial cells form this structure
10. Inner layer of skin

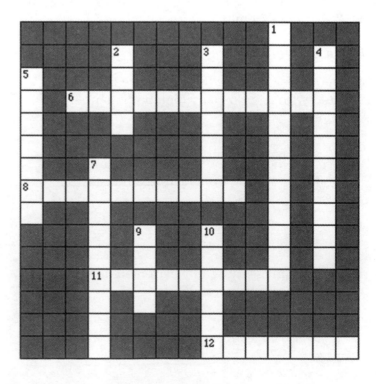

APPLYING WHAT YOU KNOW

55. Mr. Ziven was admitted to the hospital with second- and third-degree burns. Both arms, the anterior trunk, right anterior leg, and genital region were affected by the burns. The doctor quickly estimated that _____% of Mr. Ziven's body had been burned.

56. After investigating the scene of the crime, Officer Gorski announced that dermal papillae were found that would help solve the case. What did he mean?

57. Bernie is 65 and was recently diagnosed with melanoma. He finds this diagnosis difficult to believe because has lived in Alaska for the past 20 years and gets very little exposure to sun. Can you suggest a possible explanation for his diagnosis?

DID YOU KNOW

- Because the dead cells of the epidermis are constantly being worn and washed away, we get a new outer skin layer every 27 days.

- The average person sheds 40 pounds of skin in a lifetime.

ONE LAST QUICK CHECK

Multiple Choice—select the best answer.

58. Which of the following statements about hair follicles is true?
    a. Arrector pili muscles are associated with them.
    b. Sudoriferous glands empty into them.
    c. They arise directly from the epidermis layer of skin.
    d. All of the above are true.

59. Which of the following statements about apocrine glands is true?
    a. They can be classified as sudoriferous.
    b. They can be found primarily in armpit and genital regions.
    c. They secrete a thick substance that has a strong odor.
    d. All of the above are true.

60. Which of the following, if any, is *NOT* found in the dermis layer of the skin?
    a. nerves
    b. melanin
    c. blood vessels
    d. all of the above are found in the dermis

61. What characterizes second-degree burns?
    a. blisters
    b. swelling
    c. severe pain
    d. all of the above

62. Blackheads can result from the blockage of which of the following glands?
    a. lacrimal
    b. sebaceous
    c. ceruminous
    d. sudoriferous

63. Keratin is found in which layer of the skin?
    a. dermis
    b. epidermis
    c. subcutaneous
    d. serous

64. What is the fold of skin that hides the root of a nail called?
    a. lunula
    b. body
    c. cuticle
    d. papillae

65. Which of the following is *NOT* an important function of the skin?
    a. sense organ activity
    b. absorption
    c. protection
    d. temperature

66. Another name for the dermis is:
    a. corium.
    b. strata.
    c. subcutaneous.
    d. lunula.

67. The shedding of epithelial elements from the skin surface is called:
    a. desquamation.
    b. convection.
    c. cleavage lines.
    d. turnover.

Matching—identify the correct answer for each item.

a. fingerprint
b. pressure
c. brown pigment
d. perspiration
e. oil
f. follicle
g. little moon
h. axilla sweat glands
i. fungal infection
j. genetic inflammatory skin disorder

68. _____   melanin

69. _____   Pacinian corpuscle

70. _____   sebaceous

71. _____   hair

72. _____   lunula

73. _____   dermal papillae

74. _____   sudoriferous

75. _____   apocrine

76. _____   tinea

77. _____   psoriasis

CHAPTER 7

Skeletal Tissues

How strange we would look without our skeleton! It is the skeleton that provides the rigid, supportive framework that gives shape to our bodies. But this is just the beginning, because the skeleton also protects the organs beneath it, maintains homeostasis of blood calcium, produces blood cells, and assists the muscular system in providing movement for us.

After reviewing the microscopic structure of bone and cartilage, you will understand how skeletal tissues are formed, their differences and their importance in the human body. Your microscopic investigation will make the study of this system easier as you logically progress from this view to macroscopic bone formation and growth and visualize the structure of long bones.

Bones are classified structurally by their shape: long bones, short bones, flat bones, and irregular bones. They are also classified by the types of cells that form the bone: compact bone and cancellous, or spongy, bone. Throughout life, bone formation (ossification) and bone destruction (resorption) occur concurrently to assure a firm and comfortable framework for our bodies.

I—TYPES OF BONES

Matching—identify each structure with its corresponding description.

a. epiphysis
b. medullary cavity
c. carpal
d. articular cartilage
e. femur
f. endosteum
g. vertebra
h. diaphysis
i. patella
j. periosteum
k. scapulae

1. __F__ the thin membrane that lines the medullary cavity

2. __K__ an example of a flat bone

3. __h__ the shaft of the long bone

4. __e__ an example of a long bone

5. __d__ the thin layer that cushions jolts and blows

6. __i__ an example of a sesamoid bone

7. __j__ an attachment for muscle fibers

8. __c__ an example of a short bone

9. __a__ the end of a long bone

10. __b__ the tubelike, hollow space in the diaphysis of long bones

11. __g__ an example of an irregular bone

▷ *If you had difficulty with this section, review pages 230-232.*

II—BONE TISSUE STRUCTURE, FUNCTION, AND HOMEOSTASIS

Multiple Choice—select the best answer.

12. Which of the following is *NOT* a component of bone matrix?
    a. inorganic salts
    b. organic matrix
    c. collagenous fibers
    d. all of the above are components of bone matrix

13. Small spaces in which bone cells lie are called:
    a. lamellae.
    b. lacunae.
    c. canaliculi.
    d. interstitial lamellae.

14. The basic structural unit of compact bone is:
    a. trabeculae.
    b. cancellous bone.
    c. osteon.
    d. none of the above.

15. The cells that produce the organic matrix in bone are:
    a. chondrocytes.
    b. osteoblasts.
    c. osteocytes.
    d. osteoclasts.

16. The bones in an adult that contain red marrow include all of the following *EXCEPT*:
    a. ribs.
    b. tarsals.
    c. pelvis.
    d. femur.

17. Low blood calcium evokes a response from:
    a. calcitonin.
    b. thyroid.
    c. parathyroid hormone.
    d. none of the above.

True or false

18. __T__ Haversian canals run lengthwise, whereas Volkmann's canals run transverse to the bone.

19. __F__ Giant, multinucleate cells that are responsible for bone resorption are called *osteocytes*.

20. __T__ Bone marrow is found not only in the medullary cavities of certain long bones but also in the spaces of cancellous bone.

21. __T__ Calcitonin functions to stimulate osteoblasts and inhibit osteoclasts.

22. __f__ *Hematopoiesis* is a term referring to the formation of new Haversian systems.

23. __f__ Yellow marrow is found in almost all of the bones of an infant's body.

▷ *If you had difficulty with this section, review pages 232-238.*

III—BONE DEVELOPMENT, GROWTH, RESORPTION, AND REPAIR

Multiple Choice—select the best answer.

In Endochondral ossification

24. The primary ossification center is located at the:
    a. epiphysis.
    b. diaphysis.
    c. articular cartilage.
    d. none of the above.

25. The primary purpose of the epiphyseal plate is:
    a. mending fractures.
    b. enlarging the epiphysis.
    c. providing bone strength.
    d. lengthening long bones.

26. The epiphyseal plate is composed mostly of:
    a. chondrocytes.
    b. osteocytes.
    c. osteoclasts.
    d. none of the above.

27. Bone loss normally begins to exceed bone gain between the ages of:
    a. 30 and 35 years.
    b. 35 and 40 years.
    c. 55 and 60 years.
    d. 65 and 70 years.

28. The first step to healing a bone fracture is:
    a. callus formation.
    b. fracture hematoma formation.
    c. alignment of the fracture.
    d. collar formation.

True or false

29. _____ The addition of bone to its outer surface resulting in growth in diameter is called *appositional growth.*

30. _____ Most bones of the body are formed by intramembranous ossification. *endochondral*

31. _____ Once an individual reaches skeletal maturity, the bones undergo years of metabolic rest.

32. _____ Lack of exercise tends to weaken bones through decreased collagen formation and excessive calcium withdrawal.

33. _____ When bones reach their full length, the epiphyseal plate disappears.

▷ *If you had difficulty with this section, review pages 240-243.*

IV—CARTILAGE

Multiple Choice—select the best answer.

34. The fibrous covering of cartilage is:
    a. periosteum.
    b. perichondrium.
    c. chondroclast.
    d. none of the above.

35. The external ear, epiglottis, and the auditory tube are composed of:
    a. hyaline cartilage.
    b. fibrocartilage.
    c. elastic cartilage.
    d. none of the above.

36. Vitamin D deficiency can result in:
    a. scurvy.
    b. rickets.
    c. osteochondroma.
    d. none of the above.

True or false

37. _____ Both bone and cartilage are well-vascularized.

38. _____ The intervertebral discs are composed of fibrocartilage.

39. _____ The growth of cartilage occurs by both appositional and interstitial growth.

Labeling—label the following diagrams.

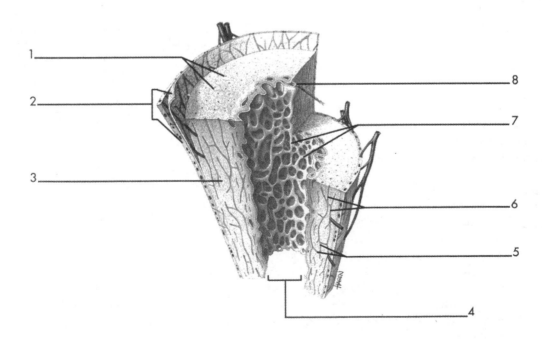

If you had difficulty with this section, review pages 244-249.

V—MECHANISMS OF DISEASE

Fill in the blanks.

40. _____ is a malignant tumor of hyaline cartilage that arises from chondroblasts.

41. _____ is the most common primary malignant tumor of skeletal tissue.

42. _____ is a common bone disease often occurring in postmenopausal women and manifesting symptoms of porous, brittle, and fragile bones.

43. _____ _____ is also known as *osteitis deformans*.

44. _____ is a bacterial infection of the bone and marrow tissue.

▷ *If you had difficulty with this section, review pages 246-249.*

Crossword Puzzle

Across
1. Ossification that replaces cartilage with bone   *endochondral*
5. Spongy bone (two words)
7. Contains osteons (two words)
9. Ends of long bone

Down
2. Bone-absorbing cell
3. Bone marrow (two words)
4. Bone-forming cell
5. Cartilage cell
6. Bone formation
8. Bone cell

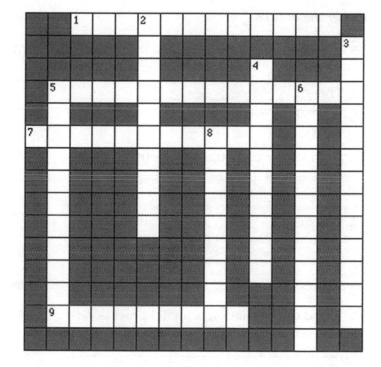

APPLYING WHAT YOU KNOW

45. Mrs. Harris is a 60-year-old white woman. She has noticed in recent years that her height has slightly decreased. Recently, she fractured her wrist in a slight fall. Which skeletal system disorder might she be suffering from? What techniques could be used to diagnose her condition? What treatments are available?

46. Mrs. Perine had advanced cancer of the bone. As the disease progressed, Mrs. Perine required several blood transfusions throughout her therapy. She asked the doctor one day to explain the necessity for the transfusions. What explanation might the doctor give to Mrs. Perine?

47. Dr. Kennedy, an orthopedic surgeon, called the admissions office of the hospital and advised them that he would be admitting a patient in the next hour with an epiphyseal fracture. Without any other information, the patient is assigned to the pediatric ward. What prompted this assignment?

48. Ms. Strickland was in an auto accident. When the surgeon described the details of the surgery to her family, he stated that he was able to "patch" her fractures. Explain what he might have meant by "patching" the fractures.

DID YOU KNOW?

- Approximately 25 million Americans have osteoporosis. Four out of five are women.

ONE LAST QUICK CHECK ✔

Fill in the blanks.

49. There are _____ types of bones.

50. The __med___ _cavity_ is the hollow area inside the diaphysis of a bone.

51. A thin layer of cartilage covering each epiphysis is the _articular_ _cartilage_.

52. The _endosteum_ lines the medullary cavity of long bones.

53. _hematopoiesis_ is used to describe the process of blood cell formation.

54. Blood cell formation is a vital process carried on in _red_ _bone_ _marrow_.

55. The _periosteum_ is a strong fibrous membrane that covers a long bone except at joint surfaces.

56. Bones may be classified by shape. Those shapes include _____, _____, _____, and _____.

57. Bones serve as the major reservoir for _Calcium_, a vital substance required for normal nerve and muscle function.

58. _____ is the most abundant type of cartilage.

Matching—identify the term with the proper selection.

a. outer covering of bone
b. dense bone tissue
c. fibers embedded in a firm gel
d. needlelike threads of spongy bone
e. ends of long bones
f. connect lacunae
g. cartilage cells
h. structural unit of compact bone
i. mature bone cells
j. ring of bone

59. __d__ trabeculae

60. __b__ compact

61. __e__ spongy

62. __a__ periosteum

63. __c__ cartilage

64. __i__ osteocytes

65. __f__ canaliculi

66. __j__ lamellae

67. __g__ chondrocytes

68. __h__ Haversian system

CHAPTER 8

Skeletal System

The skeletal system may be compared to a large 206-piece puzzle. Each bone, as with each puzzle piece, is unique in size and shape. And again, just like with a puzzle, pieces or bones are not interchangeable. They have a lock-and-key concept that allows them to fit in only one area of the skeletal frame and perform functions necessary for that location.

The skeleton is divided into two main areas: the axial skeleton and the appendicular skeleton. All of the 206 bones of the human body may be classified into one of these two areas. And although we can divide them neatly by this system, there are subtle differences that exist between a man's and a woman's skeleton that provide us with insight to the functional differences between the sexes. An understanding of the skeletal system gives us an appreciation of the complex and interdependent functions that make this system essential for maintenance of homeostasis and sustaining life.

I—DIVISIONS OF THE SKELETON

Matching—identify each term with its associated division of the skeleton.

a. axial skeleton   b. appendicular skeleton

1. _____ coccyx

2. _____ 80 bones

3. _____ 126 bones

4. _____ spinal column

5. _____ carpals

6. _____ scapulae

7. _____ auditory ossicles (ear bones)

8. _____ shoulder girdle

9. _____ skull

10. _____ clavicles

▷ *If you had difficulty with this section, review pages 256-257.*

II—THE SKULL

Multiple Choice—select the best answer.

11. The squamous suture connects which two bones?
    a. frontal and parietal
    b. parietal and temporal
    c. temporal and sphenoid
    d. sphenoid and frontal

12. The mastoid sinuses are found in which bone?
    a. frontal
    b. sphenoid
    c. parietal
    d. temporal

13. The skull bone that articulates with the first cervical vertebrae is the:
    a. occipital.
    b. sphenoid.
    c. ethmoid.
    d. none of the above.

14. A *meatus* can be described as:
    a. a large bony prominence.
    b. a shallow groove.
    c. a tubelike opening or channel.
    d. a raised, rough area.

15. Separation of the nasal and cranial cavities is achieved by the:
    a. cribriform plate of the ethmoid bone.
    b. sella turcica of the sphenoid bone.
    c. foramen magnum of the occipital bone.
    d. palatine process of the maxilla.

16. Which of the following is *NOT* a bone of the orbit?
    a. ethmoid
    b. nasal
    c. lacrimal
    d. frontal

True or false

17. _____ The sphenoid is a bone of the face.

18. _____ A specialized adaptation of the infant skull is called a *fontanel*.

19. _____ The cheek is shaped by the zygomatic, or malar, bone.

20. _____ The hyoid is one of several bones that do not articulate with any other bones.

21. _____ The external auditory meatus is located within the temporal bone.

Labeling—label the following diagrams.

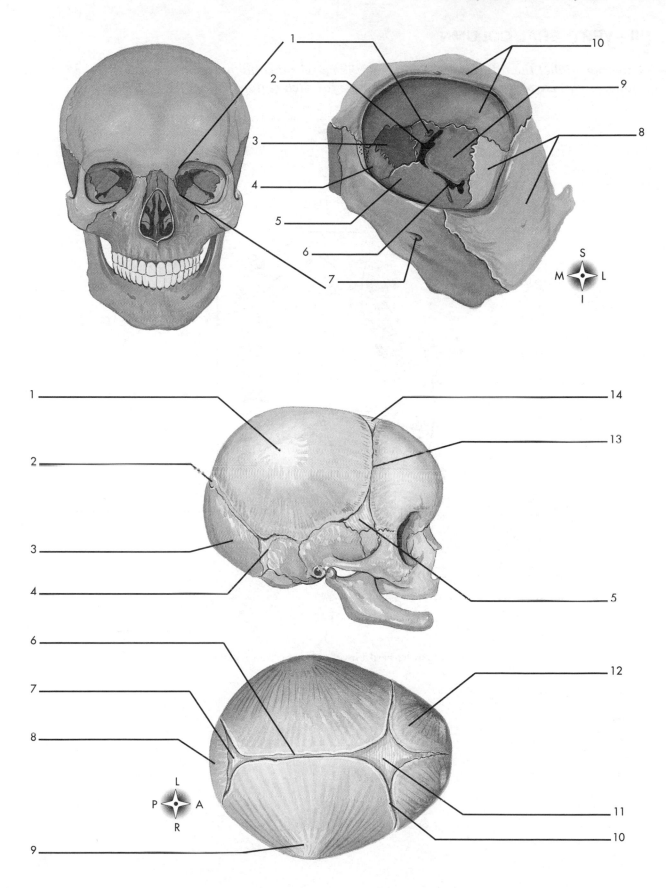

If you had difficulty with this section, review pages 256-277.

III—VERTEBRAL COLUMN

Labeling—label the following diagrams of the vertebral column. Be sure to identify the spinal regions, spinal curves, and quantity of vertebrae for each region.

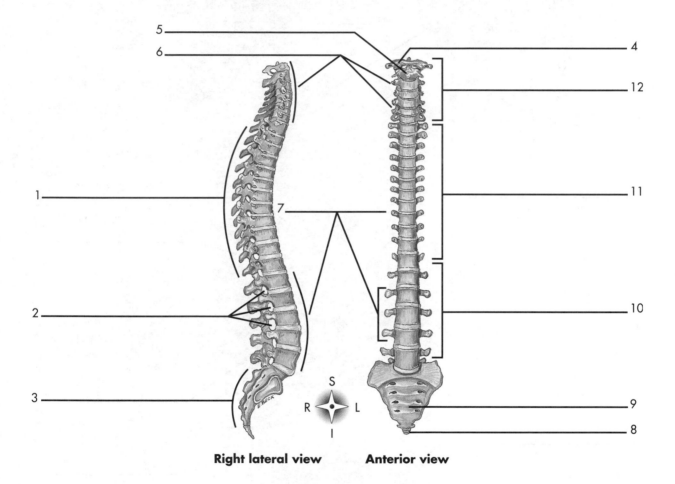

Right lateral view   **Anterior view**

Labeling—label the following images of vertebrae.

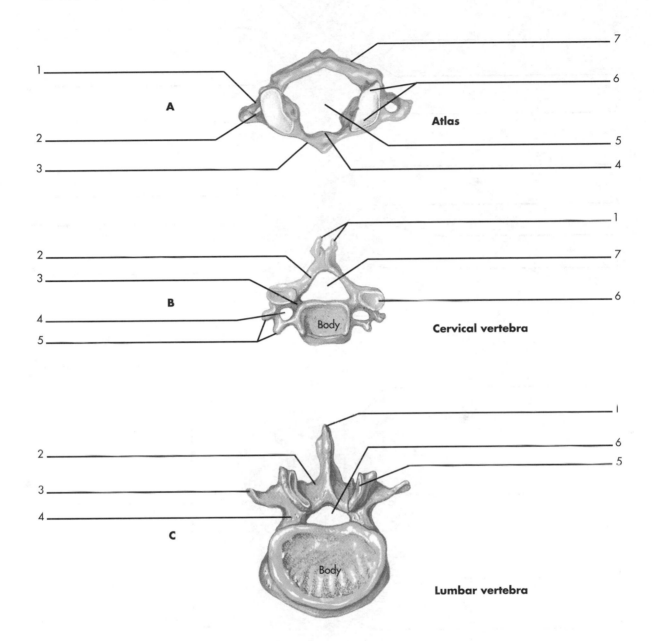

A — Atlas

B — Cervical vertebra

C — Lumbar vertebra

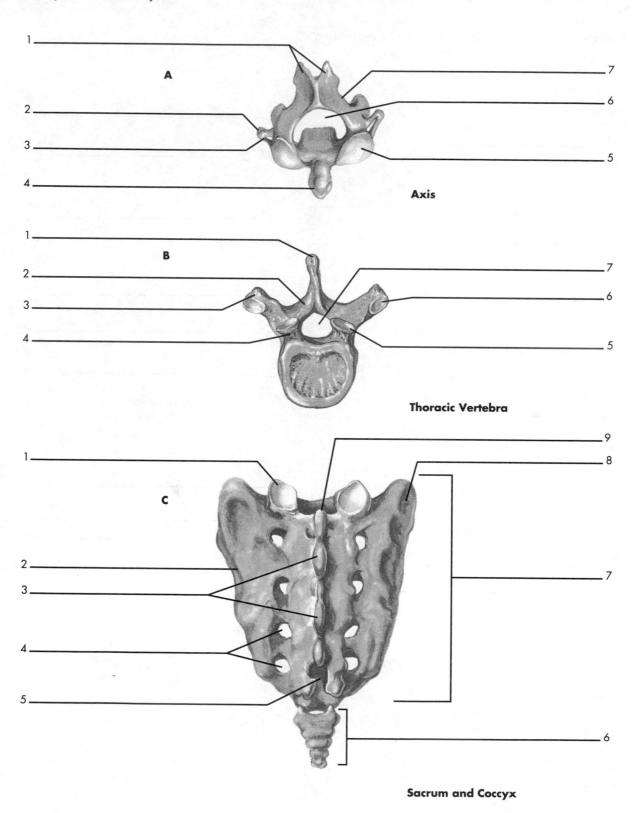

A

1
2
3
4

7
6
5

Axis

B

1
2
3
4

7
6
5

Thoracic Vertebra

C

1
2
3
4
5

9
8

7

6

Sacrum and Coccyx

▷ *If you had difficulty with this section, review pages 277-284.*

IV—STERNUM AND RIBS

Matching—identify each term with its corresponding description.

a. body
b. false ribs
c. floating ribs
d. manubrium
e. true ribs
f. xiphoid process
g. costal cartilage

22. _e_ first seven pairs of ribs that attach directly to the sternum

23. _c_ eleventh and twelfth ribs, which have no attachment to the sternum

24. _a_ middle part of the sternum

25. _d_ most superior part of the sternum

26. _f_ the blunt, cartilaginous, lower tip of the sternum

27. _b_ the five pairs of ribs that do not attach directly to the sternum

28. _g_ tissue that attaches ribs directly or indirectly to the sternum

Labeling—label the following diagrams.

▷ *If you had difficulty with this section, review pages 284-286.*

V—THE APPENDICULAR SKELETON/ UPPER EXTREMITY

Multiple Choice—select the best answer.

29. Which of the following is *NOT* part of the shoulder girdle?
    a. clavicle
    b. sternum
    c. scapula
    d. none of the above

30. The coronoid fossa is a:
    a. depression on the thumb.
    b. projection of the ulna.
    c. region on the spine.
    d. depression on the humerus.

31. The arm socket is the:
    a. coronoid fossa.
    b. olecranon fossa.
    c. coracoid process.
    d. glenoid cavity.

True or false

32. _____ The two bones that form the framework of the forearm are the radius and ulna.

33. _____ The wrist is composed of small bones called *metacarpals*.

34. _____ The medial forearm bone in the anatomical position is the ulna.

35. _____ The most evident carpal bone is the triquetrum.

Labeling—label the following diagrams.

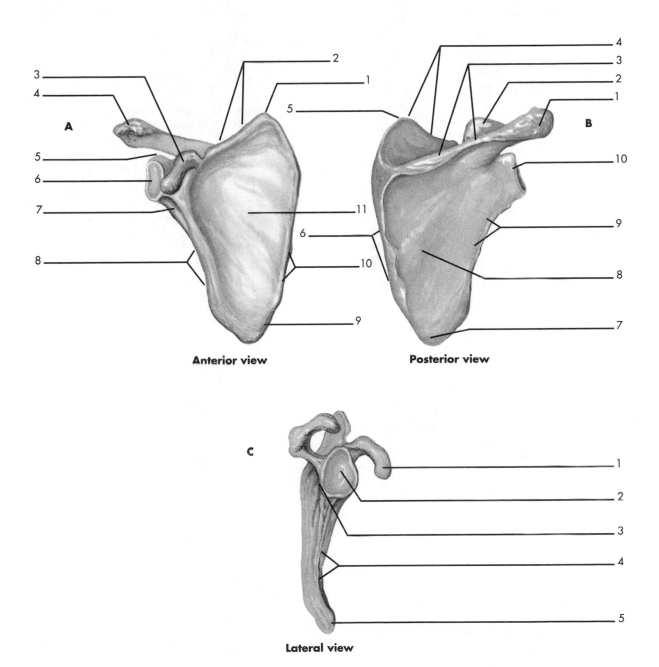

Anterior view

Posterior view

Lateral view

▶ *If you had difficulty with this section, review pages 286-289.*

VI—THE APPENDICULAR SKELETON/ LOWER EXTREMITY

Multiple Choice—select the best answer.

36. Which of the following is *NOT* one of the bones of the pelvic girdle?
    a. ilium
    b. acetabulum
    c. ischium
    d. pubis

37. The greater trochanter is a bony landmark of the:
    a. femur.
    b. tibia.
    c. pubis.
    d. ramus.

38. During childbirth, the infant passes through an imaginary plane called the:
    a. pelvic outlet.
    b. symphysis pubis.
    c. pelvic brim.
    d. ilium.

39. Which of the following is *NOT* a tarsal bone?
    a. talus
    b. cuneiform
    c. scaphoid
    d. navicular

True or false

40. _____ The largest coxal bone is the ischium.

41. _____ The most distal portion of the fibula is composed of a bony landmark called the *medial malleolus.*

42. _____ The *longitudinal arch* refers to a structure within the pelvic inlet.

43. _____ Each toe contains three phalanges.

Labeling—label the following diagrams.

▷ *If you had difficulty with this section, review pages 289-296.*

VII—SKELETAL DIFFERENCES IN MEN AND WOMEN

Matching—identify the skeletal characteristics with the appropriate gender.

a. male skeleton   b. female skeleton

44. _____ elongated forehead

45. _____ small pelvic inlet

46. _____ subpubic angle less than 90 degrees

47. _____ wide sacrum

48. _____ more massive muscle attachment sites

49. _____ more movable coccyx

▷ *If you had difficulty with this section, review page 297.*

VIII—CYCLE OF LIFE: MECHANISMS OF DISEASE

Multiple Choice—select the best answer.

50. All of the following are clinical signs and symptoms of a fracture *EXCEPT*:
    a. soft tissue edema.
    b. realignment of the bone.
    c. loss of function.
    d. pain.

51. An open fracture can be described as:
    a. a complete separation of bones.
    b. fractures in more than one area of a bone.
    c. broken bone projecting through the skin.
    d. none of the above.

True or false

52. _____   *Swayback* and *kyphosis* are syn-onymous terms.

53. _____   Normal curvature of the spine is convex posteriorly through the thoracic region and concave posteriorly through the cervical and lumbar regions.

▷ *If you had difficulty with this section, review page 299-303.*

Crossword Puzzle

Across
5. Cavity within a bone
6. Bone that is part of the spinal column
7. Encases the brain
8. Section of skeleton that includes 126 bones
10. Clavicle and scapula (two words)

Down
1. Bony cage
2. Supports the trunk (two words)
3. "Soft spot"
4. Immovable joint in skull
9. Section of skeleton that includes 80 bones

✓ APPLYING WHAT YOU KNOW

54. While playing football, Bill was involved in a tackle that caused a forced hyperextension of his elbow joint. Which skeletal structures could he have injured?

55. Amanda loves to wear extremely high-heeled shoes. How does this affect the weight distribution onto the bones of her feet? Which skeletal structures are at risk of being damaged?

DID YOU KNOW?

• The bones of the hands and feet make up more than half of the total 206 bones of the body.

• The bones of the middle ear are mature at birth.

• The skeleton of an average 160-pound body weighs about 29 pounds.

ONE LAST QUICK CHECK ✔

Circle the one that does NOT belong.

56. cervical	thoracic	coxal	coccyx
57. pelvic girdle	ankle	wrist	axial
58. frontal	occipital	maxilla	sphenoid
59. scapula	pectoral girdle	ribs	clavicle
60. malleus	vomer	incus	stapes
61. ulna	ilium	ischium	pubis
62. carpal	phalanges	metacarpal	ethmoid
63. ethmoid	parietal	occipital	nasal
64. anvil	atlas	axis	cervical

Matching—identify the bone with its marking.
There may be more than one correct answer.

a. mastoid
b. pterygoid process
c. foramen magnum
d. sella turcica
e. mental foramen
f. conchae
g. xiphoid process
h. glenoid cavity
i. olecranon process
j. ischium
k. acetabulum
l. symphysis pubis
m. ilium
n. greater trochanter
o. medial malleolus
p. calcaneus
q. acromion process
r. frontal sinuses
s. coronoid process
t. tibial tuberosity

65. _____ occipital

66. _____ sternum

67. _____ coxal

68. _____ femur

69. _____ ulna

70. _____ temporal

71. _____ tarsals

72. _____ sphenoid

73. _____ ethmoid

74. _____ scapula

75. _____ tibia

76. _____ frontal

77. _____ mandible

CHAPTER 9

Articulations

W e conclude our study of bones with a chapter on joints, or articulations. A joint, or articulation, is a point of contact between bones. Sitting, walking, and running are just a few examples of movements that would not be possible without the successful functioning of articulations. Joints also permit us to lift heavy objects and perform fine motor skills such as needlepoint. The unusual and unique shape and size of articulations are responsible for the variety and degree of motion that we expect from our body.

Joints may be classified according to structure (fibrous and cartilaginous) or according to function (synarthrosis—immovable; amphiarthrosis—slightly movable; diarthrosis—freely movable). Proper functioning of articulations is necessary for us to adapt to our environment with controlled, smooth, and pain-free movements.

I—CLASSIFICATION OF JOINTS

Multiple Choice—select the best answer.

1. The articulation between the root of a tooth and the alveolar process of the mandible or maxilla is called the:
   a. suture.
   b. gomphosis.
   c. synchondrosis.
   d. symphysis.

2. Immovable joints are called:
   a. synarthroses.
   b. amphiarthroses.
   c. diarthroses.
   d. none of the above.

3. The radioulnar articulation is classified as which type of articulation?
   a. syndesmosis
   b. synchondrosis
   c. symphysis
   d. diarthrosis

4. The most movable joints in the body are:
   a. symphyses.
   b. sutures.
   c. synovial joints.
   d. synchondroses.

5. An example of a symphysis is:
   a. the articulation between the pubic bones.
   b. the articulation between the bodies of adjacent vertebrae.
   c. both a and b.
   d. none of the above.

6. The inner surface of the joint capsule is lined with:
   a. bursae.
   b. a joint cavity.
   c. periosteum.
   d. synovial membrane.

7. The joint that allows for the widest range of movement is a _____ joint.
   a. gliding
   b. saddle
   c. ball and socket
   d. hinge

8. An example of a pivot joint is the:
   a. first metacarpal articulating with the trapezium.
   b. humerus articulating with the trapezium.
   c. interphalangeal joints.
   d. head of the radius articulating with the ulna.

True or false

9. ___T___ *Diarthrosis* and *synovial joint* refer to basically the same structure.

10. ___F___ The elbow joint is a ball and socket joint.

11. ___T___ The ability to oppose the fingers and thumb is achieved by a saddle joint.

12. ___T___ *Articulation* and *joint* are synonymous terms.

13. _____ Diarthrotic joints are the least common type of joint in the body.

14. _____ There are several examples of suture articulations throughout the entire body.

15. ___F___ Menisci are composed of hyaline cartilage.

16. ___T___ The shoulder joint is a ball and socket joint.

Matching—identify each joint or description with its corresponding classification.

a. amphiarthroses
b. diarthroses
c. synarthroses

17. ___A___ joint between bodies of vertebrae

18. ___A___ symphysis pubis

19. ___B___ hip joint

20. _____ fibrous joint

21. ___C___ immovable joint

22. _____ cartilaginous joint

23. _____ thumb

24. ___C___ joints between skull bones

25. ___b___ freely movable joint

26. ___b___ synovial joint

27. ___a___ slightly movable joint

28. _____ the most prevalent type of joint in the body

Matching—identify each joint with its corresponding functional classification.

a. ball and socket
b. condyloid
c. gliding
d. hinge
e. pivot
f. saddle

29. ___d___ elbow

30. ___c___ joints between facets of adjacent vertebrae

31. _____ ellipsoidal

32. _____ dens of axis/atlas joint

33. ___d___ knee joint

34. _____ least movable group of the synovial joints

35. ___a___ hip joint

36. ___a___ shoulder joint

37. _____ joint between first metacarpal and trapezium

Labeling—label the structures of the synovial joint on the following diagram.

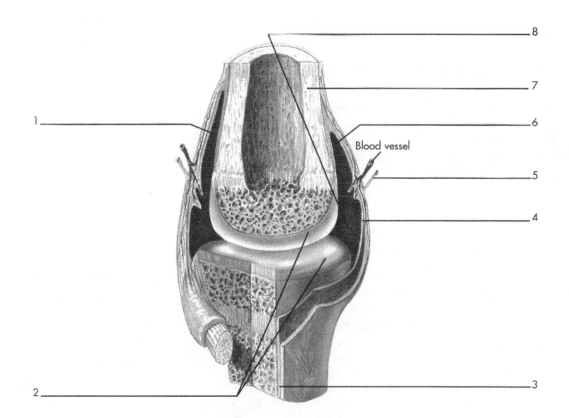

Blood vessel

▷ *If you had difficulty with this section, review pages 312-316.*

II—REPRESENTATIVE SYNOVIAL JOINTS

Multiple Choice—select the best answer.

38. The glenoid labrum is associated with which joint?
    a. hip
    b. knee
    c. shoulder
    d. vertebral

39. Perhaps the strongest ligament in the body is the:
    a. rotator cuff.
    b. iliofemoral.
    c. pubofemoral.
    d. intertrochanteric.

40. The largest and most complex joint of the body is the:
    a. shoulder.
    b. knee.
    c. hip.
    d. ankle.

41. The anterior cruciate ligament of the knee connects the:
    a. anterior tibia with the posterior femur.
    b. posterior tibia with the anterior femur.
    c. anterior fibula with the posterior femur.
    d. anterior fibula with anterior femur.

42. Vertebral bodies are connected by:
    a. the anterior longitudinal ligament.
    b. the posterior longitudinal ligament.
    c. the ligamentum flavum.
    d. both a and b.

43. Protrusion of the nucleus pulposus through the annulus fibrosus results in:
    a. bursitis.
    b. housemaid's knee.
    c. herniated disk.
    d. none of the above.

44. The medial and lateral menisci are:
    a. ligaments.
    b. cartilage.
    c. bursae.
    d. none of the above.

45. "Joint mice" are structurally:
    a. impinged bursae.
    b. loose pieces of synovial membrane.
    c. loose pieces of articular cartilage.
    d. cracks in the articular cartilage.

Labeling—label the following diagrams of synovial joints.

Shoulder joint.

Hip joint.

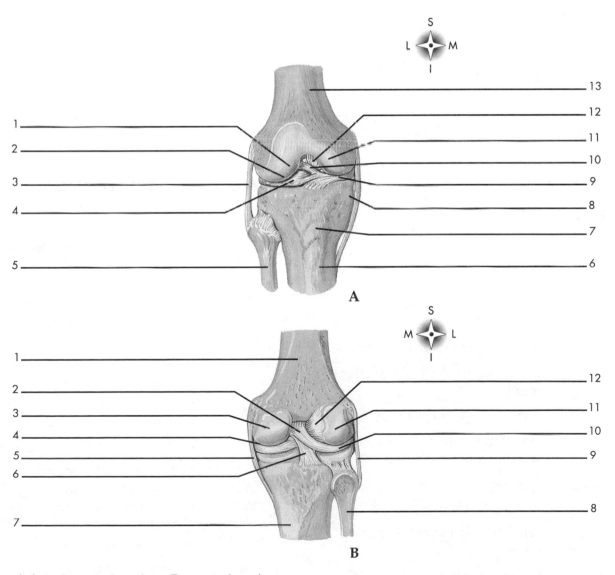

Knee joint. A, anterior view. **B,** posterior view.

1
2
3
4
5

10
9
8
7
6

S
A ✦ P
I

Vertebrae and their ligaments.

▷ *If you had difficulty with this section, review pages 317-330 and 338.*

III—TYPES AND RANGE OF MOVEMENT AT SYNOVIAL JOINTS

Matching—identify each term with its corresponding definition or description.

a. plantar flexion
b. extension
c. abduction
d. hyperextension
e. goniometer
f. rotation
g. flexion
h. inversion
i. depression
j. adduction

46. _____ instrument that measures ROM

47. __C__ lifting the arms away from the midline

48. __f__ turning the head as to say "no"

49. __g__ elbow movement, as when lifting weights during a "bicep curl"

50. __b__ increasing joint angle

51. __d__ moving beyond extension

52. __a.__ causes extension of the leg as a whole

53. __h__ turning sole of foot inward

54. _____ opening your mouth

55. __j__ bringing fingers together

▷ *If you had difficulty with this section, review pages 330-336.*

IV—MECHANISMS OF DISEASE

Fill in the blanks.

56. _____ is an imaging technique that allows a physician to examine the internal structure of a joint without the use of extensive surgery.

57. The most common noninflammatory joint disease is _____ or

_____ _____

_____.

58. A general name for many different inflammatory joint diseases is _____.

59. A metabolic type of inflammatory arthritis is_____ _____.

60. An acute musculoskeletal injury to the ligamentous structure surrounding a joint and disrupting the continuity of the synovial membrane is a _____.

▷ *If you had difficulty with this section, review pages 337-341.*

Crossword Puzzle

Across

3. Immovable joint in skull
7. Cartilaginous joint
8. Fibrous joint

Down

1. Articular disks
2. Joint
4. Synovial joint
5. A joint where fibrocartilage connect two bones
6. Pillowlike structure found between synovial joints

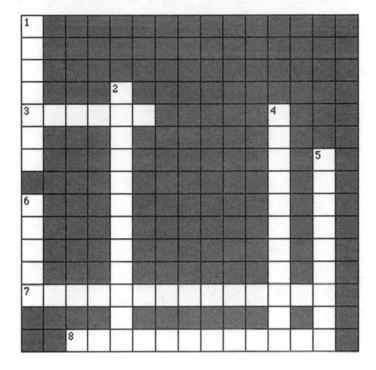

APPLYING WHAT YOU KNOW

61. Lowell is afflicted with severely inflamed joints—arthritis. If he is suffering from the chronic systemic version of this disease, what kind of symptoms would he be experiencing? Which joints are most likely involved and what is the most likely cause?

62. Sam is suffering from a type of arthritis associated with excess blood levels of uric acid. What type of arthritis is this? What symptoms might he experience, which joints would be affected, and how is this form of arthritis treated?

DID YOU KNOW

- The average person uses the leg joints to walk an average of 115,000 miles during his or her lifetime.

ONE LAST QUICK CHECK

Circle the correct answer.

63. Freely movable joints are (amphiarthroses or diarthroses).

64. The sutures in the skull are (synarthrotic or amphiarthrotic).

65. All (diarthrotic or amphiarthrotic) joints have a joint capsule, a joint cavity, and a layer of cartilage over the ends of the two joining bones.

66. (Ligaments or tendons) grow out of periosteum and attach two bones together.

67. The (articular cartilage or epiphyseal cartilage) cushions surfaces of bones.

68. Gliding joints are the (least movable or most movable) of the diarthrotic joints.

69. The knee is the (largest or smallest) joint.

70. Hinge joints allow motion in (2 or 4) directions.

71. The saddle joint at the base of each of our thumbs allows for greater (strength or mobility).

72. When you rotate your head, you are using a (gliding or pivot) joint.

True or false

73. __F__ A uniaxial joint is a synovial joint.

74. __F__ Joints identified as synchondroses are synovial joints.

75. _____ Inflammation of the bursa is referred to as *pleurisy*.

76. _____ The main bursa of the shoulder joint is the subdeltoid bursa.

77. __T__ Angular movements change the size of the angle between articulating bones.

78. __T__ Pronation is a circular movement.

79. __F__ Gliding movements are the most complex of movements.

80. __F__ Protraction is an angular movement.

81. _____ Juvenile rheumatoid arthritis is more common in boys.

82. _____ The knee joint has a "baker's dozen," or 13, bursae which serve as protective pads around it.

CHAPTER **10**

Anatomy of the Muscular System

The muscular system is often referred to as the "power system," and rightfully so, because it is this system that provides the force necessary to move the body and perform organic functions. Just as an automobile relies on the engine to provide motion, the body depends on the muscular system to perform both voluntary and involuntary types of movements. The power of this system is impressive indeed, for if we were able to direct all of our muscles in one direction, it is estimated that we would have the power to move 25 tons.

Over 600 skeletal muscles constitute 40–50% of our body weight. They are attached snugly over the skeletal frame to shape and mold the contours of our body. And while memorizing the names and locations of skeletal muscles appears to be an overwhelming task, it is comforting to learn that muscles are named and categorized quite simply. Classification and identification are focused upon location, function, shape, direction of fibers, number of heads or divisions, or points of attachment. This chapter assists you in understanding the structure of skeletal muscles and the logical approach to muscle recognition.

I—SKELETAL MUSCLE STRUCTURE

Multiple Choice—select the best answer.

1. An entire skeletal muscle is covered by a coarse sheath called:
   a. endomysium.
   b. perimysium.
   c. epimysium.
   d. aponeurosis.

2. Muscles that are arranged like the feathers in a plume are described as:
   a. parallel.
   b. convergent.
   c. sphincter.
   d. pennate.

3. An aponeurosis is:
   a. broad and flat.
   b. tube-shaped.
   c. featherlike.
   d. none of the above.

4. Antagonists are muscles that:
   a. oppose prime movers.
   b. facilitate prime movers.
   c. stabilize muscles.
   d. directly perform movements.

5. A fixed point about which a rod moves is called a:
   a. lever.
   b. bone.
   c. belly.
   d. fulcrum.

6. In first-class levers the:
   a. fulcrum is between the pull and load.
   b. load is between the fulcrum and force.
   c. force is between the fulcrum and load.
   d. load and force are equal.

True or false

7. __F__ The origin of a muscle is the point of attachment that moves when the muscle contracts.

8. __T__ Skeletal muscles usually act in groups rather than individually.

9. __T__ *Prime mover* and *agonist* are synonymous.

10. _____ The optimum angle of pull of a muscle is generally parallel to the long axis of the bone.

11. _____ Tipping the head back, as in looking up at the sky, is an example of a first-class lever.

▷ *If you had difficulty with this section, review pages 348-352.*

II—HOW MUSCLES ARE NAMED

Matching—identify each muscle with the appropriate characteristic.

a. location
b. function
c. shape
d. direction of fibers
e. number of heads
f. points of attachment
g. size of muscle

12. _____ deltoid

13. _____ brachialis

14. _____ sternocleidomastoid

15. _____ quadriceps

16. _____ gluteus maximus

17. _____ adductor

18. _____ rectus

▷ *If you had difficulty with this section, review pages 356-357.*

III—IMPORTANT SKELETAL MUSCLES: MUSCLES OF THE FACE AND NECK

Matching—identify each muscle with its appropriate body movement.

a. buccinator
b. corrugator supercilii
c. epicranius
d. orbicularis oculi
e. pterygoids
f. sternocleidomastoid

19. __b__ wrinkling the forehead vertically

20. __e__ grating the teeth during mastication

21. __a__ smiling

22. __c__ raising the eyebrows

23. __f__ flexing the head

24. __d__ closing the eyes

Labeling—label the following diagrams.

Facial muscles: (A) lateral view

Facial muscles: (B) anterior view

▷ *If you had difficulty with this section, review pages 358-362.*

IV—IMPORTANT SKELETAL MUSCLES: TRUNK MUSCLES

True or false

25. _____ The external oblique compresses the abdomen.

26. _____ The rectus abdominis flexes the trunk.

27. _____ The levator ani closes the anal canal.

28. _____ The external intercostals function to elevate the ribs.

29. _____ The coccygeus muscles and levator ani form most of the pelvic floor.

Labeling—label the following diagrams.

Muscles of the thorax.

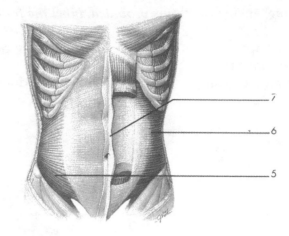

Muscles of the trunk and abdominal wall.

▷ *If you had difficulty with this section, review pages 356-370.*

V—IMPORTANT SKELETAL MUSCLES: UPPER LIMB MUSCLES

Multiple Choice   select the best answer.

30. All of the following are rotator cuff muscles *EXCEPT:*
    a. deltoid.
    b. infraspinatus.
    c. supraspinatus.
    d. teres minor.

31. The muscle that shrugs the shoulders is the:
    a. sternocleidomastoid.
    b. deltoid.
    c. trapezius.
    d. pectoralis minor

32. The posterior arm muscle that extends the forearm is the:
    a. triceps brachii.
    b. triceps surae.
    c. brachialis.
    d. biceps brachii.

33. The olecranon process of the ulna is a site of insertion for the:
    a. biceps brachii.
    b. brachialis.
    c. brachioradialis.
    d. triceps brachii.

True or false

34. _____ Intrinsic muscles of the hand originate on the forearm and insert on the metacarpals.

35. _____ Carpal tunnel syndrome affects the median nerve.

36. _____ The deltoid is a good example of a multifunction muscle.

37. _____ The pectoralis major flexes the upper arm.

38. _____ The biceps brachii is an extensor muscle.

Labeling—using the terms provided, label the following illustrations.

levator scapulae	seventh cervical vertebra	trapezius
serratus anterior	teres major	pectoralis minor
rhomboideus major	latissimus dorsi	subscapularis
teres minor	rhomboideus minor	

Muscles acting on the shoulder girdle.

Labeling—using the terms provided, label the following illustration.

subscapularis
acromion process
coracoid process
greater tubercle

intertubercular (bicipital)
groove
teres minor
humerus

supraspinatus
lesser tubercle
infraspinatus
clavicle

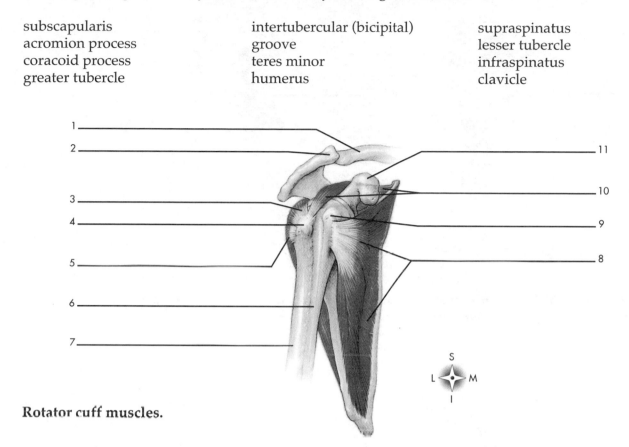

Rotator cuff muscles.

Labeling—label the following illustrations.

Twelfth thoracic
vertebra

Muscles that move the upper arm.

Muscles of the upper arm.

Labeling—on the following illustrations, label the muscles that act on the forearm. Also label the origin and insertion point of each muscle.

Muscles that act on the forearm.

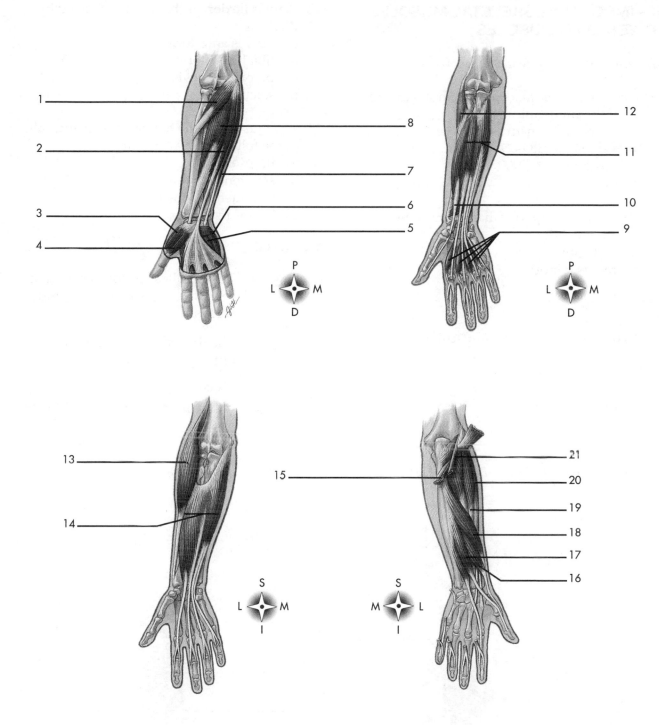

Muscles of the forearm.

▷ *If you had difficulty with this section, review pages 356 and 370-376.*

VI—IMPORTANT SKELETAL MUSCLES: LOWER LIMB MUSCLES

Multiple Choice—select the best answer.

39. The muscles of quadriceps femoris include all of the following *EXCEPT:*
    a. vastus intermedius.
    b. vastus medialis.
    c. vastus lateralis.
    d. vastus femoris.

40. The anterior superior iliac spine is the site of origin for the:
    a. sartorius.
    b. rectus femoris.
    c. gracilis.
    d. iliacus.

41. A common site for intramuscular injections is the:
    a. gluteus maximus.
    b. gluteus minimus.
    c. gluteus medius.
    d. tensor fasciae latae.

42. Plantar flexion of the foot is achieved by the:
    a. tibialis anterior.
    b. tibialis posterior.
    c. peroneus brevis.
    d. soleus.

43. The muscles of the hamstrings include all of the following *EXCEPT* the:
    a. iliopsoas.
    b. semitendinosus.
    c. semimembranosus.
    d. biceps femoris.

True or false

44. __T__ The Achilles tendon is common to both the gastrocnemius and soleus.

45. _____ The iliopsoas is composed solely of the psoas major and the iliacus.

46. _____ The vastus intermedius originates on the posterior surface of the femur.

Labeling—label the following illustrations.

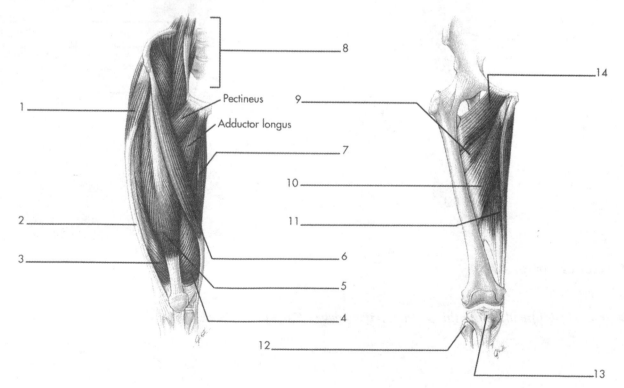

Pectineus

Adductor longus

Muscles of the upper leg.

Muscles of the lower leg.

 If you had difficulty with this section, review pages 381-388.

Crossword Puzzle

Across
3. Attachment that does not move
7. Agonist (two words)
8. Opposes prime mover

Down
1. Rigid bar free to turn about its fulcrum
2. Contracts at the same time as the prime mover
4. Attachment that moves
5. Joint stabilizer
6. Maintaining optimal body position

APPLYING WHAT YOU KNOW

47. Mr. Lynch spends hours typing on his computer. As of late, he is experiencing weakness, pain, and tingling in the palm and radial aspect of the hand. What condition may he be experiencing? Which anatomical structures are most likely involved? Which options for treatment are available?

48. The nurse was preparing an injection for Mrs. Tatakis. The amount to be given was 2 ml. What area of the body will the nurse most likely select for the injection?

49. Al is analyzing the musculature involved in the athletes he coaches. Today he is observing a basketball player executing a jump shot. Which muscles are involved at the hips, knees, and ankles as the athlete jumps? Which muscles are involved at the shoulders, elbows, and wrists as the athlete shoots the basketball?

DID YOU KNOW?

- The muscles of the hand begin to grow rapidly between 6 and 7 years of age.

- A cat has 32 muscles in each ear.

ONE LAST QUICK CHECK ✔

Matching—choose the proper function(s) for the muscles listed. Muscles may have more than one answer.

a. flexor
b. extensor
c. abductor
d. adductor
e. rotator
f. dorsiflexor or plantar flexor

50. _____   deltoid

51. _____   tibialis anterior

52. _____   gastrocnemius

53. _____   biceps brachii

54. _____   gluteus medius

55. _____   soleus

56. _____   iliopsoas

57. _____   pectoralis major

58. _____   gluteus maximus

59. _____   triceps brachii

60. _____   sternocleidomastoid

61. _____   trapezius

62. _____   gracilis

Matching—identify the term with the appropriate description.

a. contracts simultaneously with the prime mover
b. attachment to the more movable bone
c. functions as joint stabilizer
d. attachment to more stationary bone
e. when contracting, directly opposes prime mover

63. __d__   origin

64. __b__   insertion

65. __a__   synergist

66. __e__   antagonist

67. __c__   fixator

CHAPTER 11

Physiology of the Muscular System

Although the muscular system has several functions, the primary purpose is to provide movement or power. Muscles produce power by contracting. The ability of a large muscle or muscle group to contract depends on the ability of microscopic muscle fibers to contract within the larger muscle. An understanding of these microscopic muscle fibers will assist you as you progress in your study to the larger muscles and muscle groups.

Three types of muscles provide us with a variety of motions. When skeletal or voluntary muscles contract, they provide movement of bones, heat production, and posture. Smooth muscles are found throughout the viscera of our body and assist with involuntary functions such as peristalsis. Cardiac muscle is the third and final type of muscle. It lines the wall of the heart and promotes the pumping action necessary for life. Our muscles must be used to keep the body healthy and in good condition. Scientific evidence keeps pointing to the fact that the proper use and exercise of muscles may prolong life. An understanding of the structure and function of the muscular system may, therefore, add quality and quantity to our lives.

I—FUNCTION OF SKELETAL MUSCLE TISSUE

Multiple Choice—select the best answer.

1. Which of the following is *NOT* a general function of muscle tissue?
   a. movement
   b. protection
   c. heat production
   d. posture

2. The skeletal muscle fiber characteristic of excitability directly results in these cells being capable of:
   a. responding to nerve signals.
   b. shortening.
   c. returning to resting length after contracting.
   d. producing heat.

3. The correct order of arrangement of skeletal muscle cells, from largest to smallest, is:
   a. fiber, myofibril, myofilament.
   b. myofibril, myofilament, fiber.
   c. myofilament, myofibril, fiber.
   d. fiber, myofilament, myofibril.

4. Sarcoplasmic reticulum is:
   a. a system of transverse tubules that extend at a right angle to the long axis of the cell.
   b. a segment of the myofibril between two successive Z lines.
   c. a unique name for the plasma membrane of a muscle fiber.
   d. none of the above.

5. Which of the following are myofilament proteins?
   a. troponin
   b. tropomyosin
   c. a and b
   d. none of the above

6. The contractile unit of a myofibril is the:
   a. sarcomere.
   b. triad.
   c. sarcolemma.
   d. cross bridge.

7. The chief function of the T tubule is to:
   a. provide nutrients to the muscle fiber.
   b. allow the fiber to contract.
   c. allow the electrical signal to move deep into the cell.
   d. allow the generation of new muscle fibers.

8. Myosin heads are also called:
   a. cross bridges.
   b. motor endplates.
   c. synapses.
   d. motor neurons.

9. During muscle contraction, Ca⁺⁺ is released from the:
   a. synaptic cleft.
   b. mitochondria.
   c. sarcoplasmic reticulum.
   d. sarcoplasm.

10. The region of a muscle fiber where a motor neuron connects to the muscle fiber is called the:
    a. synaptic vesicle.
    b. motor end-plate.
    c. H band.
    d. none of the above.

True or false

11. _____ The thick myofilament is made up of myosin.

12. _____ Skeletal muscle has a poor ability to stretch.

13. _____ A T tubule sandwiched between sacs of sarcoplasmic reticulum is called a *codon.*

14. _____ Actin, troponin, and tropomyosin are present on the thin myofilament.

15. _____ The I band resides within a single sarcomere.

16. _____ Rigor mortis is caused because of the lack of ATP to "turn off" muscle contraction.

17. _____ The cell membrane of a muscle fiber is called the *sarcoplasmic reticulum.*

18. _____ Anaerobic respiration is the first choice of the muscle cell for the production of ATP.

19. _____ During rest, excess oxygen molecules in the sarcoplasm are attracted to a large protein molecule called *myoglobin.*

20. _____ Anaerobic respiration results in the formation of an incompletely catabolized molecule called *lactic acid.*

Labeling—using the terms provided, label the structure of skeletal muscle on the following diagrams.

sarcomere	Z line	Z disk
sarcoplasmic reticulum	Fascicle	thick filament
myofibril	fascia	tendon
thin filament	muscle fiber	endomysium
bone	perimysium	muscle
T tubule	epimysium	

Labeling—using the terms provided, label the following diagrams.

sarcoplasm	Schwann cell	myelin sheath
synaptic vesicle	motor endplate	synaptic cleft
sarcoplasmic reticulum	sarcomere	myofibril
motor neuron fiber	sarcolemma	mitochondria
acetylcholine receptor sites	triad	T tubule

▷ *If you had difficulty with this section, review pages 396-405.*

II—FUNCTION OF SKELETAL MUSCLE ORGANS

Multiple Choice—select the best answer.

21. The principal component(s) of a motor unit is/are:
    a. one somatic motor neuron.
    b. the muscle fibers supplied by a somatic motor neuron.
    c. none of the above.
    d. both a and b.

22. The staircase phenomenon is also known as:
    a. tetanus.
    b. electromyography.
    c. wave summation.
    d. treppe.

23. Skeletal muscles are innervated by:
    a. somatic motor neurons.
    b. autonomic motor neurons.
    c. both a and b.
    d. internal stimulation.

24. Which of the following statements concerning isometric contractions is true?
    a. The length of the muscle changes.
    b. Muscle tension decreases.
    c. Joint movements are swift.
    d. Muscle length remains constant.

25. Physiological muscle fatigue is caused by:
    a. relative lack of ATP.
    b. oxygen debt.
    c. lack of will.
    d. none of the above.

26. Increase in muscle size is called:
    a. hyperplasia.
    b. atrophy.
    c. hypertrophy.
    d. treppe.

27. Endurance training is also called:
    a. isometrics.
    b. hypertrophy.
    c. aerobic training.
    d. anaerobic training.

True or false

28. _____   A muscle contracts the instant it is stimulated.

29. _____   Isotonic contraction is a contraction in which the tone or tension within a muscle remains the same, but the length of the muscle changes.

30. _____   One method of studying muscle contraction is called *myography*.

31. _____   Muscles with more tone than normal are described as *flaccid*.

Labeling—using the terms provided, label the following illustration.

myofibrils

neuromuscular junction

nucleus

motor neuron

myelin sheath

muscle fibers

Schwann cell

▷ *If you had difficulty with this section, review pages 406-415.*

III—FUNCTION OF CARDIAC AND SMOOTH MUSCLE TISSUE

Matching—identify each muscle tissue with its corresponding characteristics.

a. cardiac muscle tissue
b. skeletal muscle tissue
c. smooth muscle tissue

32. _____ located in the walls of the digestive tract

33. _____ contains many nuclei near the sarcolemma

34. _____ voluntary

35. _____ not striated

36. _____ striated; contains a single nucleus

37. _____ a principal function: peristalsis

38. _____ has larger (in diameter) T tubules that form diads with sarcoplasmic reticulum

39. _____ principal functions: movement of bones, heat production, and posture

40. _____ contains intercalated disks

41. _____ has poorly developed sarcoplasmic reticulum

Labeling—label the following diagram of a cardiac muscle fiber.

▶ *If you had difficulty with this section, review pages 415-417.*

IV—MECHANISMS OF DISEASE

Circle the correct answer.

42. Muscle strains are characterized by (myalgia or fibromyositis).

43. Crush injuries can cause (hemoglobin or myoglobin) to accumulate in the blood and result in kidney failure.

44. A viral infection of the nerves that controls skeletal muscle movement is known as (poliomyelitis or muscular dystrophy).

45. (Muscular dystrophy or myasthenia gravis) is a group of genetic diseases characterized by atrophy of skeletal muscle tissues.

46. (Muscular dystrophy or myasthenia gravis) is an autoimmune disease in which the immune system attacks muscle cells at the neuromuscular junction.

▶ *If you had difficulty with this section, review pages 419-420.*

Crossword Puzzle

Across

1. Thick and thin
4. Smooth, sustained muscle contraction
8. "Same length"
9. Transverse structure unique to muscle cells (two words)

Down

1. Motor neuron plus the muscle fibers (two words)
2. Junction between nerve endings and muscle fibers
3. Plasma membrane of striated muscle fiber
5. Principle that states a muscle fiber will contract fully or not at all (three words)
6. "Same tension"
7. Fine subunit of muscle fiber

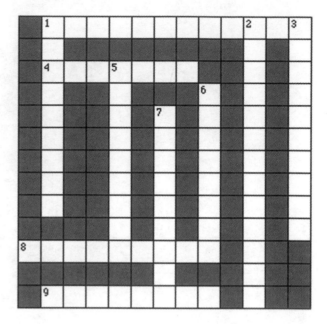

APPLYING WHAT YOU KNOW

47. Throughout Linda's life, she wanted to be a star in the 100-meter dash. However, no matter how hard she trained, she could never excel in this sport. On the other hand, she *did* achieve great success in much longer track events, especially the 10-kilometer race. Explain Linda's situation from the aspect of which skeletal muscle fiber type she may possess disproportionately by virtue of her genetics.

48. John is working in a hospital while he is studying to become a physician. One of his duties is to transport recently deceased patients to the morgue. While moving the patients onto the gurney, he is surprised to discover how stiff the bodies can be. Which physiological phenomenon is responsible for this stiffness? Exactly why is it that these muscles can temporarily display stiffness?

DID YOU KNOW

- The simple act of walking requires the use of 200 muscles in the human body.

- People who are on bed rest or totally inactive lose approximately 1% muscle strength per day.

ONE LAST QUICK CHECK

Multiple Choice—select the best answer.

49. When a muscle does not shorten and no movement results, the contraction is:
    a. isometric.
    b. isotonic.
    c. twitch.
    d. tetanic.

50. Pushing against a wall is an example of which type of contraction?
    a. isotonic
    b. isometric
    c. twitch
    d. tetanic

51. Prolonged inactivity causes muscles to shrink in mass, a condition called:
    a. hypertrophy.
    b. disuse atrophy.
    c. paralysis.
    d. muscle fatigue.

52. Muscle fibers usually contract to about _____% of their starting length.
    a. 50
    b. 60
    c. 70
    d. 80

53. Which statement is true of smooth muscle?
    a. It lines the walls of many hollow organs.
    b. It is striated.
    c. It is voluntary.
    d. There are many T tubules throughout smooth muscle.

54. What is a quick, jerky response of a given muscle to a single stimulus called?
    a. isometric
    b. lockjaw
    c. tetanus
    d. twitch

True or false

55. _____ The energy required for muscular contraction is obtained by hydrolysis of amino acids.

56. _____ A motor neuron together with the cells it innervates is called a *motor unit.*

57. _____ If muscle cells are stimulated repeatedly without adequate periods of rest, the strength of the muscle contraction will decrease, resulting in fatigue.

58. _____ The minimal level of stimulation required to cause a fiber to contract is called the *threshold stimulus.*

59. _____ Weakness of abdominal muscles can lead to a hernia.

60. _____ There are two types of smooth muscle: visceral and multiunit.

61. _____ Cardiac muscle is also known as *striated involuntary.*

62. _____ The length/tension relationship states that the maximal strength a muscle can develop is related to the length of the fibers.

63. _____ Skeletal muscles have little effect on body temperature.

CHAPTER 12

Nervous System Cells

The nervous system organizes and coordinates the millions of impulses received each day to make communication with and enjoyment of our environment possible. The functioning unit of the nervous system is the neuron. Three types of neurons exist—sensory, motor, and interneurons—which are classified according to the direction in which they transmit impulses. Nerve impulses travel over routes made up of neurons and provide the rapid communication necessary for maintaining life.

Your study of the nervous system begins with the simplest concept of impulse conduction known as the *reflex arc*. It then progresses to the more complex pathways such as divergence/convergence. An understanding of the anatomy and physiology of the nervous system cells is necessary before you progress to the complexity of this system and its multiple divisions.

I—ORGANIZATION OF THE NERVOUS SYSTEM

Matching—identify each part of the nervous system with its definition.

a. afferent division
b. autonomic nervous system
c. central nervous system
d. efferent nervous system
e. parasympathetic division
f. peripheral nervous system
g. somatic nervous system
h. sympathetic division

1. _____ consists of the brain and spinal cord

2. _____ composed of nerves arising from the brain and spinal cord

3. _____ PNS subdivision that transmits incoming information from the sensory organs to CNS

4. _____ produces the "fight or flight" response

5. _____ subdivision that carries information from the CNS to skeletal muscle

6. _____   subdivision of efferent division that transmits information to smooth muscle, cardiac muscle, and glands

7. _____   consists of all outgoing motor pathways

8. _____   coordinates the body's normal resting activities

▷ *If you had difficulty with this section, review pages 432-433.*

II—CELLS OF THE NERVOUS SYSTEM

Matching—identify each type of cell with its characteristics.

a. astrocyte
b. microglia
c. oligodendrocyte
d. Schwann cell

9. _____   has the ability of phagocytosis

10. _____   helps to form the blood-brain barrier

11. _____   produces fatty myelin sheath in PNS

12. _____   largest and most numerous of the neuroglial cells

13. _____   produces myelin sheath in CNS

14. _____   type of neuroglia that forms the neurilemma

15. _____   "star-cell"

16. _____   disorder of this cell associated with multiple sclerosis

Multiple Choice—select the best answer.

17. Which of the following are classified as nerve fibers?
    a. axon
    b. dendrites
    e. both a and c
    d. none of the above

18. Which of the following conduct impulses towards the cell body?
    a. axons
    b. dendrites
    c. Nissl bodies
    d. none of the above

19. A neuron with one axon and several dendrites is a:
    a. multipolar neuron.
    b. unipolar neuron.
    c. bipolar neuron.
    d. none of the above.

20. Which type of neuron lies entirely within the CNS?
    a. afferent
    b. efferent
    c. interneuron
    d. none of the above

21. Which sequence best represents the course of an impulse over a reflex arc?
    a. receptor, synapse, sensory neuron, motor neuron, effector
    b. effector, sensory neuron, synapse, motor neuron, receptor
    c. receptor, motor neuron, synapse, sensory neuron, effector
    d. receptor, sensory neuron, interneuron, motor neuron, effector

Labeling—label the following illustration showing the structure of a typical neuron.

1. _____
2. _____
3. _____
4. _____
5. _____
6. _____
7. _____
8. _____
9. _____
10. _____
11. _____
12. _____
13. _____   14. _____

Labeling—using the terms provided, label the following illustration of a myelinated axon.

neurilemma (sheath of Schwann cell)   myelin sheath
plasma membrane of axon   node of Ranvier
nucleus of Schwann cell   neurofibrils

Labeling—identify the classification of each type of neuron in the following illustrations.

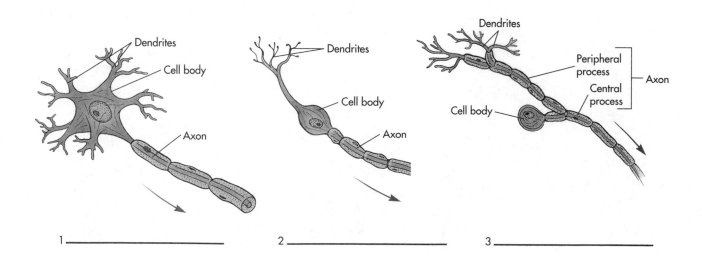

1 _____   2 _____   3 _____

Labeling—using the terms provided, label the following illustration of a reflex arc.

gray matter   cell body   white matter
interneuron   spinal nerve   synapse
sensory neuron axon   motor neuron axon   dendrite

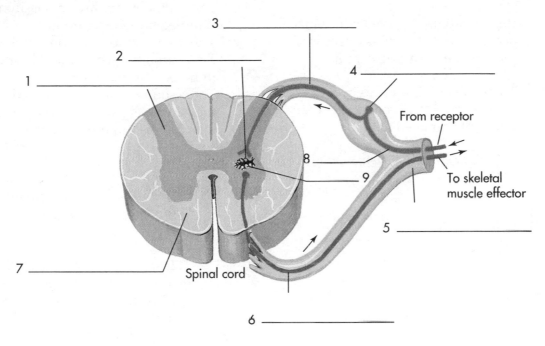

3 _____

2 _____

1 _____

From receptor

8

9

To skeletal
muscle effector

5 _____

7 _____

Spinal cord

6 _____

▷ *If you had difficulty with this section, review pages 434-443.*

III—NERVES AND TRACTS

Multiple Choice—select the best answer.

22. A complete nerve, consisting of numerous fascicles and their blood supply, is held together by a fibrous coat called the:
    a. endoneurium.
    b. perineurium.
    c. epineurium.
    d. fascicle.

23. Small, distinct regions of gray matter within the CNS are usually called:
    a. white matter.
    b. nuclei.
    c. ganglia.
    d. fascicle.

24. Nerves that contain mostly efferent fibers are called:
    a. sensory nerves.
    b. motor nerves.
    c. mixed nerves.
    d. Schwann nerves.

25. Gray matter in the CNS consists of:
    a. nerve fibers.
    b. neuroglia.
    c. axons.
    d. cell bodies.

26. Most nerves in the human nervous system are:
    a. sensory nerves.
    b. motor nerves.
    c. mixed nerves.
    d. reflex nerves.

▷ *If you had difficulty with this section, review page 443.*

IV—REPAIR OF NERVE FIBERS

True or false

27. _____   Neurons have a vast ability to re-pair themselves.

28. _____   Regeneration of nerve fibers will occur if the cell body is intact and the fibers have a neurilemma.

29. _____   There are no differences between the CNS and PNS concerning the repair of damaged fibers.

▷ *If you had difficulty with this section, review pages 443-444.*

V—NERVE IMPULSES

Multiple Choice—select the best answer.

30. Compared with the inside of the cell, the outside of most cell membranes is:
    a. positive.
    b. negative.
    c. equal.
    d. none of the above.

31. The difference in electrical charge across a plasma membrane is called:
    a. depolarization.
    b. membrane potential.
    c. both a and b.
    d. none of the above.

32. A neuron's resting membrane potential is:
    a. 70 mV.
    b. −70 mV.
    c. 30 mV.
    d. −30 mV.

33. Which of the following statements is true concerning the sodium-potassium pump?
    a. Three sodium ions are pumped out of the neuron for every two potassium ions pumped into the neuron.
    b. Two sodium ions are pumped out of the neuron for every three potassium ions pumped into the neuron.
    c. Three sodium ions are pumped out of the neuron for every three chloride ions pumped into the neuron.
    d. Three sodium ions are pumped out of the neuron for every three potassium ions pumped into the neuron.

True or false

34. _____   A membrane that exhibits a membrane potential is said to be *polarized.*

35. _____   A slight shift away from the resting membrane potential in a specific region of the plasma membrane is often called a *stimulus-gated channel.*

36. _____   Chlorine ions (Cl^-) are the dominant extracellular cations.

▷ *If you had difficulty with this section, review pages 443-447.*

VI—ACTION POTENTIAL

Multiple Choice—select the best answer.

37. During a relative refractory period:
    a. an action potential is impossible.
    b. an action potential is possible only in response to a very strong stimuli.
    c. an action potential is occurring.
    d. none of the above.

38. Voltage-gated channels are:
    a. membrane channels that close during voltage fluctuations.
    b. membrane channels that open in response to voltage fluctuations.
    c. membrane channels that are altered from an extremely high stimulus.
    d. none of the above.

39. When current leaps across an insulating myelin sheath from node of Ranvier to node of Ranvier, the type of impulse conduction is:
    a. repolarization.
    b. refraction.
    c. saltatory conduction.
    d. diffusion.

40. The larger the diameter of a nerve fiber:
    a. the slower the speed of conduction.
    b. the faster the speed of conduction.
    c. Fiber diameter does not influence speed of conduction.
    d. the more the speed fluctuates.

True or false

41. _____ *Action potential* and *nerve impulse* are synonymous.

42. _____ When repolarization has occurred, an impulse cannot be conducted.

43. _____ The action potential is an all-or-none response.

44. _____ Many anesthetics function by inhibiting the opening of sodium channels and thus blocking the initiation and conduction of nerve impulses.

▷ *If you had difficulty with this section, review pages 447-449 and 456.*

VII—SYNAPTIC TRANSMISSION

Multiple Choice—select the best answer.

45. Which of the following structures is *NOT* a main component of a chemical synapse?
    a. synaptic knob
    b. synaptic cleft
    c. synaptic process
    d. plasma membrane of postsynaptic neuron

46. A synaptic knob is located on the:
    a. synaptic cleft.
    b. axon.
    c. dendrite.
    d. cell body.

47. Which of the following is true of spatial summation?
    a. Neurotransmitters released simultaneously from several presynaptic knobs converge on one postsynaptic neuron.
    b. Simultaneous stimulation of more than one postsynaptic neuron occurs.
    c. Impulses are fired in a rapid succession by the same neuron.
    d. Speed of impulse transmission is increased when several neurotransmitters are released.

True or false

48. _____ In an adult, the nervous system is replete with both electrical synapses and chemical synapses.

49. _____ Rapid-succession stimulation of a postsynaptic neuron by a synaptic knob can have a cumulative effect over time that can result in an action potential.

50. _____ Ca^{++} ions cause the release of neurotransmitters across the synaptic cleft.

Labeling—using the terms provided, label the following illustration of a chemical synapse.

synaptic knob
stimulus-gated Na⁺ channels
presynaptic cell
synaptic cleft

postsynaptic cell action potential
voltage-gated K⁺ channels
voltage-gated Ca⁺⁺ channels

▷ *If you had difficulty with this section, review pages 450-452.*

VII—NEUROTRANSMITTERS

Multiple Choice—select the best answer.

51. Neurotransmitters are released in a synapse and bind to:
    a. presynaptic terminals.
    b. the synaptic cleft.
    c. the base of the axon.
    d. receptors on the postsynaptic terminal.

52. The main chemical classes of neurotransmitters include all of the following EXCEPT:
    a. acetylcholine.
    b. norepinephrine.
    c. amino acids.
    d. amines.

53. Which of the following is NOT an example of an amine neurotransmitter?
    a. serotonin
    b. histamine
    c. glycine
    d. dopamine

54. Severe depression can be caused by a deficit in which of the following neurotransmitters?
    a. acetylcholine
    b. amino acids
    c. amines
    d. neuropeptides

dopamine

55. Which of the following is *NOT* a catecholamine?
    a. epinephrine
    b. norepinephrine
    c. dopamine
    d. serotonin

True or false

56. _____ Many biologists now believe that neuropeptides are the most common neurotransmitters in the CNS.

57. ___T___ Cocaine produces a temporary feeling of well-being by blocking the uptake of dopamine.

▷ *If you had difficulty with this section, review pages 456-461.*

Crossword Puzzle

Across
6. Bundle of peripheral nerve fibers
7. Membrane potential of an active neuron (two words)
10. Place where signals are transmitted from one to another neuron
12. Transmits impulses toward the cell body

Down
1. Consists of a cell body, an axon, and one or more dendrites
2. _____ potential or difference in electrical charge across the plasma membrane
3. White, fatty substance
4. Supporting cell of the nervous system
5. Signal conduction route to and from the CNS (two words)
8. Center of entire nervous system (abbrev.)
9. Nerves that lie in the "periphery" (abbrev.)
11. Transmits impulses away from the cell body

VIII—MECHANISMS OF DISEASE

Fill in the blanks.

58. _____ _____ is a disorder of the nervous system that involves the glia rather than neurons.

59. _____ is a common type of brain tumor that is usually benign but may still be life-threatening.

60. A highly malignant form of astrocytic tumor is known as _____ _____.

61. Joseph Merrick, the so-called Elephant Man, suffered from _____ _____.

62. Most disorders of the nervous system cells involve _____ rather than neurons.

▷ *If you had difficulty with this section, review pages 463-464.*

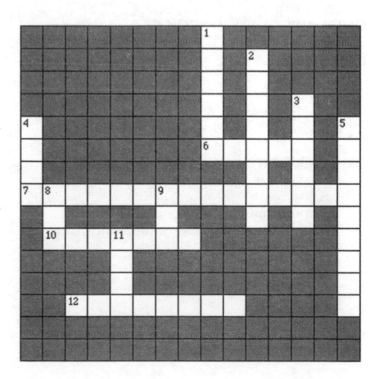

APPLYING WHAT YOU KNOW

63. Jim is experiencing muscular weakness, loss of coordination, visual impairment, and speech disturbances. Which disease of the CNS could he be experiencing? Which nervous tissue cells are most likely involved? What specifically occurs to both the neurons and neuroglia of the CNS? What are the possible treatments and what are the theories as to the cause of this disease?

64. John is a professional football player who, upon a severe compressing blow to the head, lost the ability to move his lower body. He was rushed to the hospital where the doctors suspected crushing and bruising to the spinal cord. What are the chances of the damaged nervous tissue repairing itself?

DID YOU KNOW

• In the adult human body, there are 46 miles of nerves.

ONE LAST QUICK CHECK

Circle the correct answer.

65. A synaptic knob is a tiny bulge at the end of the (presynaptic or postsynaptic) neuron's axon.

66. Acetylcholine is an example of a (neurotransmitter or protein molecule receptor).

67. Neurotransmitters are chemicals that allow neurons to (communicate or reproduce) with one another.

68. Neurotransmitters are distributed (randomly or specifically) into groups of neurons.

69. Endorphins and enkephalins are neurotransmitters that inhibit conduction of (fear or pain).

70. Unipolar neurons are always (sensory or motor) neurons.

71. In the peripheral nervous system, small regions of gray matter are known as (nuclei or ganglia).

72. The distal tips of axons form branches called (telodendria or axon hillock).

Matching—select the best choice for the following words and insert the correct letter in the blanks.

a. neurons   b. neuroglia

73. _____ axon

74. _____ supporting cells

75. _____ astrocytes

76. _____ sensory

77. _____ conduct impulses

78. _____ forms the myelin sheath around central nerve fibers

79. _____ phagocytosis

80. _____ efferent

81. _____ multiple sclerosis

82. _____ multipolar

CHAPTER 13

Central Nervous System

Approximately one hundred billion neurons make up the brain. Everything we are and everything we hope to become are centered in this structure which is about the size of a small bowling ball. Our personality, communication skills, memory, and sensations depend upon the successful functioning of the brain. We are still in the infancy of our knowledge of this unique organ as it still holds many mysteries for scientists to uncover. We are fascinated by the fact that although all pain is felt and interpreted in the brain, the brain itself has no pain sensation—even when cut! This simple example illustrates the complexity of the brain and some of the challenges ahead in identifying and understanding its capabilities for our body.

The central nervous system (CNS) is made up of the spinal cord and brain. The spinal cord provides access to and from the brain by means of ascending and descending tracts. In addition, the spinal cord functions as the primary reflex center of the body. The brain consists of the brain stem, cerebellum, diencephalon, and cerebrum. These areas provide the extraordinary network necessary to receive, interpret, and respond to most of our impulses. Your study of the CNS will give you an appreciation of the complex mechanisms necessary to perform your daily tasks.

I—COVERINGS OF THE BRAIN AND SPINAL CORD

Multiple Choice—select the best answer.

1. From superficial to deep, which is the correct order of location of the meninges?
   a. dura mater, arachnoid membrane, pia mater
   b. pia mater, arachnoid membrane, dura mater
   c. arachnoid membrane, pia mater, dura mater
   d. dura mater, pia mater, arachnoid membrane

2. The falx cerebri separates the:
   a. two hemispheres of the cerebellum.
   b. cerebellum from the cerebrum.
   c. two hemispheres of the cerebrum.
   d. dura mater from the arachnoid.

3. The cerebrospinal fluid resides in the:
   a. epidural space.
   b. subarachnoid space.
   c. subdural space.
   d. piarachnoid space.

4. The layer of the meninges that serves as the inner periosteum of the cranial bones is the:
   a. pia mater.
   b. arachnoid membrane.
   c. dura mater.

Labeling—label the coverings of the brain on the following diagram.

▶ *If you had difficulty with this section, review page 472.*

II—CEREBROSPINAL FLUID

Multiple Choice—select the best answer.

5. Formation of the cerebrospinal fluid occurs mainly in the:
   a. cerebral aqueduct.
   b. superior sagittal sinus.
   c. choroid plexuses.
   d. median foramen.

6. The lateral ventricles are located within the:
   a. cerebrum.
   b. cerebellum.
   c. spinal cord.
   d. none of the above.

7. CSF is absorbed into the venous blood via the:
   a. cisterna magna.
   b. choroid plexus.
   c. falx cerebri.
   d. arachnoid villus.

8. Cerebrospinal fluid is *NOT* found in the:
   a. central canal.
   b. subarachnoid space.
   c. third ventricle.
   d. subdural space.

True or false

9. _____ The four large, fluid-filled spaces within the brain are called *ventricles.*

10. _____ Interference of the CSF circulation, causing the fluid to accumulate in the subarachnoid space, is referred to as *external hydrocephalus.*

Labeling—label the following illustration of the fluid spaces of the brain.

Labeling—label the following illustrations depicting the flow of cerebrospinal fluid and the layers of the brain.

▷ *If you had difficulty with this section, review pages 475-479.*

III—THE SPINAL CORD

Matching—identify each ascending, or sensory, tract with its corresponding function.

a. lateral spinothalamic tract
b. anterior spinothalamic tract
c. fasciculi gracilis and cuneatus
d. spinocerebellar tract

11. _____   transmits impulses of crude touch and pressure

12. _____   transmits impulses of subconscious kinesthesia

13. _____   transmits impulses of crude touch, pain, and temperature

14. _____   transmits impulses of discriminating touch and kinesthesia

Matching—identify each descending, or motor, tract with its corresponding function.

a. lateral corticospinal tract
b. anterior corticospinal tract
c. reticulospinal tract
d. tactospinal tract
e. rubrospinal tract

15. _____   transmits impulses that control voluntary movement of muscles on the same side of the body

16. _____   facilitates head and neck movement related to visual reflexes

17. _____   helps maintain posture during skeletal muscle movements

18. _____   transmits impulses that control voluntary movement of muscles on the opposite side of the body

19. _____   transmits impulses that coordinate body movements and maintenance of posture

Labeling—match each spinal cord term with its corresponding number in the following illustration.

_____ white matter

_____ anterior median fissure

_____ cauda equina

_____ spinal nerve

_____ posterior column

_____ gray matter

_____ lumbar enlargement

_____ cervical enlargement

_____ end of spinal cord

_____ anterior column

_____ central canal

_____ dorsal nerve root

_____ filum terminale

_____ lateral column

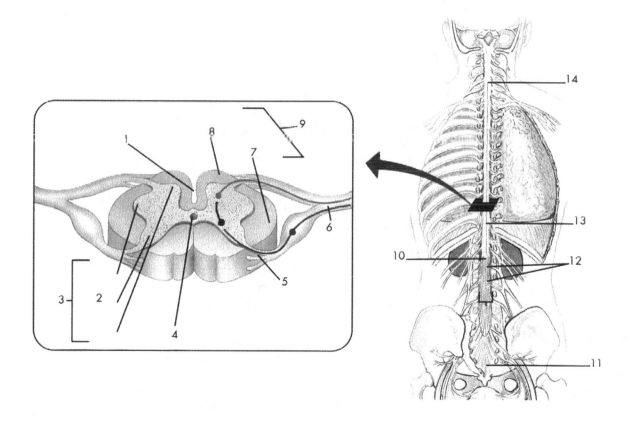

Labeling—using the terms provided, label the major tracts of the spinal cord on the following diagram.

fasciculus gracilis	rubrospinal	anterior spinocerebellar
anterior spinothalamic	reticulospinal	spinotectal
lateral spinothalamic	fasciculus cuneatus	vestibulospinal
lateral corticospinal	posterior spinocerebellar	tectospinal
anterior corticospinal		

 If you had difficulty with this section, review pages 479-482.

IV—THE BRAIN

Multiple Choice—select the best answer.

20. Which of the following is *NOT* a part of the brainstem?
    a. medulla oblongata
    b. hypothalamus
    c. pons
    d. midbrain

21. Which of the following is *NOT* a component of the midbrain?
    a. cerebral peduncles
    b. corpora quadrigemina
    c. superior colliculi
    d. all of the above are part of the midbrain

22. The internal white matter of the cerebellum is the:
    a. arbor vitae.
    b. vermis.
    c. peduncle.
    d. none of the above.

23. The part of the brain that secretes releasing hormones is the:
    a. thalamus.
    b. hypothalamus.
    c. medulla.
    d. pons.

24. Regulation of the body's biological clock and production of melatonin is performed by the:
    a. pons.
    b. thalamus.
    c. cerebellum.
    d. pineal body.

25. The central sulcus divides the:
    a. temporal lobe and parietal lobe.
    b. cerebrum into two hemispheres.
    c. frontal lobe and parietal lobe.
    d. occipital lobe and parietal lobe.

26. The part of the cerebrum integral to consciousness is:
    a. Broca's area.
    b. the reticular activating system.
    c. the limbic system.
    d. the insula.

27. The two cerebral hemispheres are connected by the:
    a. corpus callosum.
    b. mammillary body.
    c. hippocampus.
    d. central sulcus.

28. Emotions involve the functioning of the cerebrum's:
    a. Broca's area.
    b. limbic system.
    c. reticular activating system.
    d. caudate nucleus.

29. The type of brain wave associated with deep sleep is:
    a. delta.
    b. beta.
    c. alpha.
    d. theta.

True or false

30. ___T___ The cerebellum is the second largest portion of the brain.

31. ___F___ Functions of the cerebellum include language, memory, and emotions.

32. ___F___ The vomiting reflex is mediated by the cerebellum.

33. ___T___ The shallow grooves of the cerebrum are called *sulci*.

34. ___T___ The islands of gray matter inside the hemispheres of the cerebrum are called the *basal ganglia*.

Labeling—label the following illustration of the left hemisphere of the cerebrum.

Labeling—label the functional areas of the cerebral cortex on the following illustration.

▷ *If you had difficulty with this section, review pages 482-501.*

IV—SOMATIC SENSORY AND MOTOR PATHWAYS

Multiple Choice—select the best answer.

35. Which of the following is *NOT* a pathway that produces sensations of touch and pressure?
    a. medial lemniscal system
    b. spinothalamic pathway
    c. rubrospinal tract

36. Axons from the anterior gray horn of the spinal cord terminate in:
    a. cerebral cortex.
    b. sensory receptors.
    c. skeletal muscle.
    d. none of the above.

37. Absence of reflexes is indicative of injury to:
    a. lower motor neurons.
    b. upper motor neurons.
    c. lower sensory neurons.
    d. upper sensory neurons.

True or false

38. _____ Poliomyelitis results in flaccid paralysis via destruction of anterior horn neurons.

39. _____ Extrapyramidal tracts are very simple pyramidal tracts.

▷ *If you had difficulty with this section, review pages 501-504.*

VI—MECHANISMS OF DISEASE

Matching—identify each disorder with its corresponding definition.

a. Alzheimer disease
b. cerebrovascular accident
c. epilepsy
d. Huntington disease

40. __D__ an inherited form of dementia in which the symptoms first appear between 30 and 40 years of age

41. __B__ a hemorrhage from or cessation of blood flow to the cerebral vessels, which destroys neurons

42. __A__ a degenerative disease that affects memory, generally developing during the middle to late adult years and causing characteristic lesions in the cortex

43. __C__ recurring or chronic seizure episodes involving sudden bursts of abnormal neuron activity

▷ *If you had difficulty with this section, review pages 505-506.*

Crossword Puzzle

Across

1. _____ formation consisting of gray and white matter located in medulla
4. Largest division of the brain
8. Contains midbrain, pons, and medulla
9. Helps maintain normal body temperature
10. Electroencephalogram (abbrev.)
11. Cerebrospinal fluid (abbrev.)
12. Second largest part of the brain

Down

2. "Emotional brain" (two words)
3. "Between brain"
5. Part of diencephalon
6. Large, fluid-filled spaces within the brain
7. Membranous coverings of brain

APPLYING WHAT YOU KNOW

44. Baby Dania was born with an excessive accumulation of cerebrospinal fluid in the ventricles. A catheter was placed in the ventricle and the fluid was drained by means of a shunt into the circulating bloodstream. What condition does this medical history describe? *hydrocephalus*

45. Julius is exhibiting loss of memory, increasingly limited attention span, deteriorating motor control, and changes in his personality. What is the general term that can be used to describe his condition? What specific condition may he be suffering from?

DID YOU KNOW

- The short-term memory capacity for most people is between five and nine items or digits. This is one reason that phone numbers were kept to seven digits (not including the area code).

- The soft mass of the adult brain is motionless. Though it consumes up to 24% of the blood's oxygen supply, it does not grow, divide, or contract.

ONE LAST QUICK CHECK ✔

Matching—select the best choice and insert the correct letter in the answer blank.

a. SPECT
b. MRI
c. CT
d. hemiplegia
e. cerebral palsy
f. EEG
g. AIDS
h. CVA
i. dementia
j. PET

46. _____ stroke

47. _____ paralysis

48. _____ a crippling disease that involves permanent, nonprogressive damage to motor control areas of the brain

49. _____ an imaging technique for the brain that involves scanning the head with a revolving x-ray generator

50. _____ a scanning method that determines the functional characteristics of the brain by introducing a radioactive substance into the blood supply of the brain

51. _____ used to visualize blood flow in the brain

52. _____ a scanning method that uses a magnetic field to induce brain tissues to emit radio waves

53. _____ measurement of electrical activity of the brain

54. _____ characteristic of Alzheimer disease

55. _____ caused by the HIV virus

Multiple Choice—select the best answer.

56. The portion of the brain stem that joins the spinal cord to the brain is the:
    a. pons.
    b. cerebellum.
    c. diencephalon.
    d. hypothalamus.
    e. medulla.

57. Which one of the following is *NOT* a function of the brain stem?
    a. conducts sensory impulses from the spinal cord to the higher centers of the brain
    b. conducts motor impulses from the cerebrum to the spinal cord
    c. controls heartbeat, respiration, and blood vessel diameter
    d. contains centers for speech and memory

58. Which one of the following is *NOT* part of the diencephalon?
    a. cerebrum
    b. thalamus
    c. hypothalamus
    d. pineal gland

59. Which one of the following parts of the brain helps in the association of sensations with emotions, as well as aiding in the arousal or alerting mechanism?
    a. pons
    b. hypothalamus
    c. cerebellum
    d. thalamus *epithalamus*
    e. none of the above is correct

60. Which one of the following is *NOT* a function of the cerebrum?
    a. language
    b. consciousness
    c. memory
    d. conscious awareness of sensations
    e. all of the above are functions of the cerebrum

61. The area of the cerebrum responsible for the perception of sound lies in the _____ lobe.
    a. frontal
    b. temporal
    c. occipital
    d. parietal

62. Visual perception is located in the _____ lobe.
    a. frontal
    b. temporal
    c. occipital
    d. parietal

63. Which one of the following is *NOT* a function of the cerebellum?
    a. maintains equilibrium
    b. helps produce smooth, coordinated movements
    c. helps maintain normal posture
    d. associates sensations with emotions

64. The largest section of the brain is the:
    a. cerebellum.
    b. pons.
    c. cerebrum.
    d. midbrain.

65. Which statement is false?
    a. The spinal cord performs two general functions.
    b. A lumbar puncture is performed to withdraw cerebrospinal fluid.
    c. The cardiac, vasomotor, and respiratory control centers are called the *vital centers*.
    d. REM sleep is almost always a dreamless sleep.

66. Parkinson disease is a disease of the:
    a. myelin.
    b. axons.
    c. neuroglia.
    d. cerebral nuclei.

CHAPTER 14

Peripheral Nervous System

While you concentrate on this chapter, your body is performing a multitude of functions. Fortunately for us, the beating of the heart, digestion of food, breathing, and most of our day-to-day processes do not require our supervision or thought. They function automatically, and the division of the nervous system that regulates these functions is known as the *autonomic nervous system.*

The autonomic nervous system is a division of the peripheral nervous system (PNS). There are two functional divisions of the PNS—the afferent (sensory) division and the efferent (motor) division. The efferent division is divided into the somatic nervous system which is responsible for voluntary motor responses and the autonomic nervous system which is responsible for involuntary motor responses. The autonomic nervous system consists of two divisions called the *sympathetic system* and the *parasympathetic system.* The sympathetic system functions as an emergency system and prepares us for "fight or flight." The parasympathetic system dominates control of many visceral effectors under normal everyday conditions. Together, these two divisions regulate the body's automatic functions in an effort to assist with the maintenance of homeostasis. Your understanding of this chapter will alert you to the functions and complexity of the peripheral nervous system and the "automatic pilot" of your body—the autonomic system.

I—SPINAL NERVES

Multiple Choice—select the best answer.

1. Which of the following is an *incorrect* statement?
   a. There are 7 cervical nerve pairs.
   b. There are 12 thoracic nerve pairs.
   c. There are 5 lumbar nerve pairs
   d. All of the above are correct statements.

2. The spinal root that has a noticeable swelling is the:
   a. ventral root.
   b. anterior root.
   c. dorsal root.
   d. none of the above.

3. The dorsal root ganglion contains:
   a. sensory neuron cell bodies.
   b. motor neuron cell bodies.
   c. both sensory neuron and motor neuron cell bodies.
   d. motor neuron fibers.

4. The phrenic nerve innervates the:
   a. spleen.
   b. diaphragm.
   c. chest muscles.
   d. none of the above.

5. The femoral nerve arises from the:
   a. lumbar plexus.
   b. sacral plexus.
   c. coccygeal plexus.
   d. brachial plexus.

True or false

6. ___T___ The lower end of the spinal cord is called the *cauda equina*.

7. ___T___ There are 31 pairs of spinal nerves, all of which are composed of both motor and sensory fibers.

8. ___F___ Herpes zoster is a unique bacterial infection that almost always affects the skin of a single dermatome.

9. ___F___ *Dermatome* is a term referring to a skeletal muscle group innervated by motor neuron axons from a given spinal nerve.

10. ___T___ The brachial plexus is found deep within the shoulder.

Labeling—using the terms provided, label the spinal nerves on the following illustration.

cervical plexus   coccygeal nerve   cervical nerves   lumbar nerves
brachial plexus   cervical vertebrae   cauda equina   sacrum
thoracic vertebrae   sacral nerves   thoracic nerves   dura mater
coccyx   lumbar vertebrae

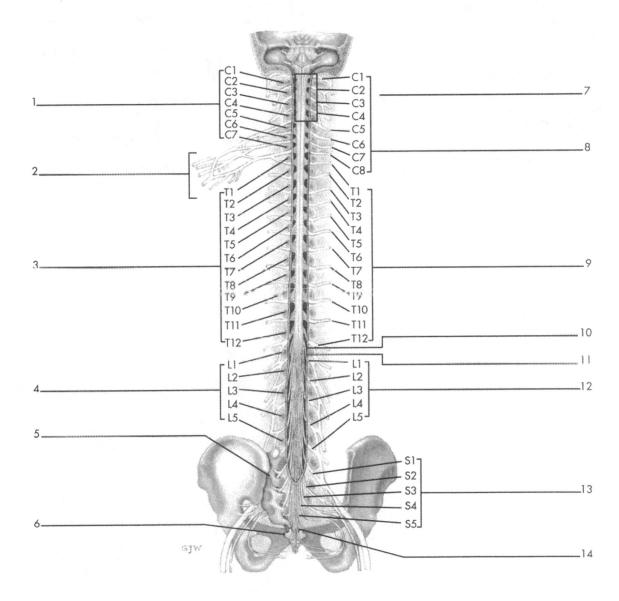

▷ *If you had difficulty with this section, review pages 516-525.*

II—CRANIAL NERVES

Matching—identify each cranial nerve with its corresponding function.

a. olfactory
b. optic
c. oculomotor
d. trochlear
e. trigeminal
f. abducens
g. facial
h. vestibulocochlear
i. glossopharyngeal
j. vagus
k. accessory
l. hypoglossal

11. _____ facial expressions

12. _____ sense of smell

13. _____ peristalsis

14. _____ hearing and balance

15. _____ vision

16. _____ chewing

17. _____ swallowing

18. _____ regulation of pupil size

19. _____ innervation of the superior oblique muscle of the eye

20. _____ abduction of the eye

21. _____ tongue movements

22. _____ shoulder movements

Labeling—identify the cranial nerves by matching each term with its corresponding number in the following illustration.

_10_ glossopharyngeal nerve (IX)

_12_ olfactory nerve (I)

_4_ abducens nerve (VI)

_6_ vestibulocochlear nerve (VIII)

_7_ vagus nerve (X)

_9_ hypoglossal nerve (XII)

_11_ trigeminal nerve (V)

_3_ oculomotor nerve (III)

_5_ facial nerve (VII)

_1_ trochlear nerve (IV)

_8_ accessory nerve (XI)

_2_ optic nerve (II)

▷ *If you had difficulty with this section, review pages 525-533.*

III—SOMATIC MOTOR NERVOUS SYSTEM

Multiple Choice—select the best answer.

23. Somatic effectors are:
    a. smooth muscle.
    b. skeletal muscle.
    c. cardiac muscle.
    d. glands.

24. When the outer sole of the foot is stimulated, a normal infant will extend the great toe. This is called the:
    a. Babinski reflex.
    b. plantar reflex.
    c. tendon reflex.
    d. corneal reflex.

25. Which is the neurotransmitter in a somatic motor pathway?
    a. acetylcholine
    b. amines
    c. amino acids
    d. neuropeptides

Labeling—label the neural pathway involved in the patellar reflex on the following illustration.

 If you had difficulty with this section, review pages 533-534.

IV—AUTONOMIC NERVOUS SYSTEM

Multiple Choice—select the best answer.

26. Somatic motor and autonomic pathways share all of the following *EXCEPT*:
    a. direction of impulse conduction.
    b. effectors located outside the CNS.
    c. number of neurons between the CNS and effector.
    d. acetylcholine as a possible neurotransmitter.

27. Within the sympathetic chain ganglion, the preganglionic fiber may:
    a. synapse with a sympathetic postganglionic neuron.
    b. send an ascending branch through the sympathetic trunk.
    c. pass through chain and synapse in a collateral ganglion.
    d. all of the above.

28. Beta receptors bind with:
    a. acetylcholine.
    b. norepinephrine.
    c. toxin muscarine.
    d. none of the above.

29. Which of the following is *NOT* an example of sympathetic stimulation?
    a. constriction of the bronchioles
    b. decreased secretion of the pancreas
    c. constriction of the urinary sphincters
    d. dilation of skeletal muscle blood vessels

30. "Fight or flight" physiological changes include all of the following *EXCEPT*:
    a. increased conversion of glycogen to glucose.
    b. constriction of respiratory airways.
    c. increased perspiration.
    d. dilation of blood vessels in skeletal muscles.

True or false

31. __F__ Conduction of autonomic effectors requires only one efferent neuron.

32. __T__ Many autonomic effectors are dually innervated.

33. __T__ The sympathetic division is also called the *thoracolumbar division*.

34. __F__ The sympathetic division is the dominant controller of the body at rest.

35. __T__ Sympathetic responses are usually widespread, involving many organ systems at once.

Labeling—using the terms provided, label the following diagram of autonomic conduction paths.

sympathetic ganglion
postganglionic neuron axon
sympathetic trunk
sympathetic rami

collateral ganglion
preganglionic sympathetic neuron axon
somatic motor neuron axon

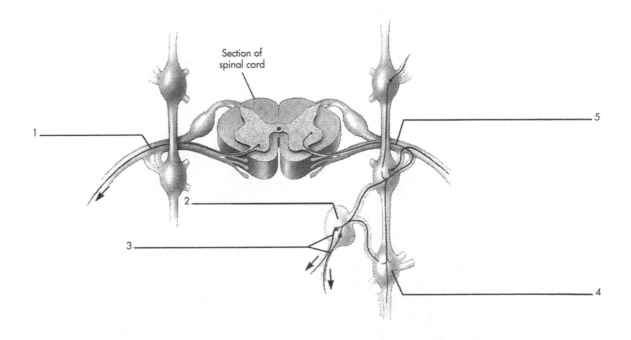

▶ *If you had difficulty with this section, review pages 535-544.*

Crossword Puzzle

Across

2. Division that serves as the "fight or flight" reaction
4. Along with autonomic nerve and plexuses, makes up efferent autonomic pathway
5. Division that controls most autonomic effectors most of the time
8. Action that results from a nerve impulse passing over a reflex arc
9. Large branches of spinal nerve
10. "Horse's tail" (two words)

Down

1. "Skin section"
2. 31 pairs (two words)
3. Trochlear is an example (two words)
6. A spinal nerve may also be called this (two words)
7. Complex network formed by ventral rami of most spinal nerves

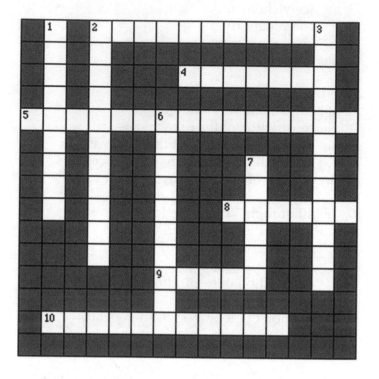

APPLYING WHAT YOU KNOW

36. Cara experiences great anxiety before her college final exams. As the professor distributes the exam, she experiences a classic "fight or flight" reaction. Which division of the autonomic nervous system is responsible for this phenomenon? Which body systems are affected and how do they respond? What is Cara's risk of chronic exposure to such stress?

37. Greg is under great stress from trying to advance in his career, pursue graduate school, and raise two small children. After a particularly stressful event, he noticed a burning sensation in his axillary and pectoral regions. Days later he experienced an eruption of red swollen plaques in the same area. What condition is he experiencing? What is the name of the responsible pathogen? Why did he experience the symptoms that he did? What may be the reason that the pathogen was capable of breaching his immune system?

DID YOU KNOW?

- The human brain continues sending out electrical wave signals for up to 37 hours after death.

- The brain begins to lose cells at a rate of 50,000 per day by age 30.

- Eighty percent of the average human brain is water.

ONE LAST QUICK CHECK

Matching—identify the term with the proper selection.

a. division of ANS
b. tissues to which autonomic neurons conduct impulses
c. voluntary actions
d. regulates body's involuntary effectors
e. efferent neurons that make up the ANS
f. conduct impulses between the spinal cord and a ganglion

38. _____ autonomic nervous system

39. _____ autonomic neurons

40. _____ preganglionic neurons

41. _____ visceral effectors

42. _____ sympathetic system

43. _____ somatic nervous system

Multiple Choice—select the best answer.

44. Dendrites and cell bodies of sympathetic preganglionic neurons are located in the:
    a. brain stem and sacral portion of the spinal cord.
    b. sympathetic ganglia.
    c. gray matter of the thoracic and upper lumbar segments of the spinal cord.
    d. ganglia close to effectors.

45. Which of the following is *NOT* correct?
    a. Sympathetic preganglionic neurons have their cell bodies located in the lateral gray column of certain parts of the spinal cord.
    b. Sympathetic preganglionic axons pass along the dorsal root of certain spinal nerves.
    c. There are synapses within sympathetic ganglia.
    d. Sympathetic responses are usually widespread, involving many organs.

46. Another name for the parasympathetic nervous system is:
    a. thoracolumbar.
    b. craniosacral.
    c. visceral.
    d. ANS.
    e. cholinergic.

47. Which statement is *NOT* correct?
    a. Sympathetic postganglionic neurons have their dendrites and cell bodies in sympathetic ganglion or collateral ganglia.
    b. Sympathetic ganglions are located in front of and at each side of the spinal column.
    c. Separate autonomic nerves distribute many sympathetic postganglionic axons to various internal organs.
    d. Very few sympathetic preganglionic axons synapse with postganglionic neurons.

Matching—select the correct response and insert the letter in the answer blank.

a. sympathetic control
b. parasympathetic control

48. __b__ constricts pupils

49. __a__ "goose pimples"

50. __a__ increases sweat secretion

51. __b__ increases secretion of digestive juices and insulin

52. __a__ constricts blood vessels

53. __b__ slows heartbeat

54. __a__ relaxes bladder

55. __a__ increases epinephrine secretion

56. __b__ increases peristalsis

57. __b__ accommodates lens for near vision

Matching—select the best choice for the following words and insert the correct letter in the answer blank.

a. cranial nerves   b. spinal nerves

58. _____   12 pairs

59. _____   dermatome

60. _____   vagus

61. _____   shingles

62. _____   31 pairs

63. _____   optic

64. _____   C1

65. _____   plexus

CHAPTER 15

Sense Organs

Consider this scene for a moment. You are walking along a beautiful beach watching the sunset. You notice the various hues and are amazed at the multitude of shades that cover the sky. The waves are melodious as they splash along the shore and you wiggle your feet with delight as you sense the warm, soft sand trickling between your toes. You sip on a soda and then inhale the fresh salt air as you continue your stroll along the shore. It is a memorable scene, but one that would not be possible without the assistance of your sense organs. The sense organs pick up messages that are sent over nerve pathways to specialized areas in the brain for interpretation. They make communication with and enjoyment of the environment possible. The visual, auditory, tactile, olfactory, and gustatory sense organs not only protect us from danger but also add an important dimension to our daily pleasures of life. Your study of this chapter will give you an understanding of another one of the systems necessary for homeostasis and survival.

I—SENSORY RECEPTORS

Multiple Choice—select the best answer.

1. Which of the following is *NOT* a general sense?
   a. touch
   b. taste
   c. temperature
   d. pain

2. Which of the following is *NOT* a true statement?
   a. Mechanoreceptors are activated by stimuli that "deform" the receptor.
   b. Taste and smell are examples of chemoreceptors.
   c. Photoreceptors respond to light stimuli.
   d. Thermoreceptors are activated by pressure.

3. Which of the following structures is a disc-shaped nerve ending that is responsible for discerning light touch?
   a. Merkel discs
   b. pacinian corpuscles
   c. nociceptors
   d. Golgi tendon receptors

4. Which of the following is *NOT* a proprio-
   ceptor?
   a. muscle spindle
   b. root hair plexus
   c. Golgi tendon receptor
   d. all of the above are proprioceptors

5. Proprioceptors:
   a. function in relation to movements and
      body position.
   b. are superficial.
   c. are receptors for touch, pain, heat, and
      cold.
   d. are widely distributed throughout the
      skin.

True or false

6. _____ Mechanoreceptors are activated
   by a change in temperature.

7. _____ Free nerve endings are the simplest, most common, and most
   widely distributed sensory receptors.

8. _____ Somatic sense receptors located
   in muscles and joints are called
   visceroreceptors.

9. _____ Golgi tendon receptors are stimulated by excessive muscle contraction.

10. _____ Exteroceptors are often called *cu-
    taneous receptors* because of their
    placement in the skin.

▷ *If you had difficulty with this section, review
pages 554-560.*

II—THE SENSE OF SMELL AND THE SENSE OF TASTE

Multiple Choice—select the best answer.

11. Olfactory receptors and taste buds are:
    a. thermoreceptors.
    b. chemoreceptors.
    c. nociceptors.
    d. mechanoreceptors.

12. Olfactory epithelium consists of:
    a. epithelial support cells.
    b. basal cells.
    c. cilia.
    d. all of the above.

13. All of the following are primary taste sen-
    sations *EXCEPT*:
    a. sweet.
    b. sour.
    c. spicy.
    d. bitter.

14. Nerve impulses responsible for the sensa-
    tion of taste are carried in all of the follow-
    ing cranial nerves *EXCEPT*:
    a. VII.
    b. VIII.
    c. IX.
    d. X.

True or false

15. ___T___ Olfaction requires the chemical
    response of a dissolved substance
    for a stimulus.

16. _____ The olfactory receptor cells lie in
    an excellent position functionally
    to smell delicate odors.

17. _____ The transmission pathway for
    olfactory sensations is as follows:
    olfactory cilia, olfactory bulb, ol-
    factory tract, thalamic, and olfac-
    tory centers of the brain.

18. _____ The tip of the tongue reacts best
    to bitter taste.

Labeling—label the midsagittal section of the nasal area on the following illustration.

 If you had difficulty with this section, review pages 560-564.

III—SENSE OF HEARING AND BALANCE: THE EAR

Multiple Choice—select the best answer.

19. Which of the following is a structure of the middle ear?
    a. incus
    b. oval window
    c. cranial nerve VII
    d. vestibule

20. The auditory tube connects the:
    a. inner ear and cranial nerve VIII.
    b. middle ear and the auditory ossicles.
    c. middle ear and the nasopharynx.
    d. oval window and the round window.

21. The only structure of the inner ear concerned with hearing is the:
    a. utricle.
    b. saccule.
    c. semicircular canals.
    d. cochlear duct.

22. Dynamic equilibrium depends upon the functioning of the:
    a. organ of Corti.
    b. crista ampullaris.
    c. both a and b.
    d. none of the above.

23. The neuronal pathway of hearing begins at the:
    a. vestibular nerve.
    b. cochlear nerve.
    c. vestibulocochlear nerve.
    d. cranial nerve VII.

24. The passageway leading to the tympanic membrane is the:
    a. external auditory meatus.
    b. auditory tube.
    c. eustachian tube.
    d. oval window.

25. The sense organ(s) responsible for the sense of balance is/are located in the:
    a. vestibule.
    b. cochlea.
    c. semicircular canals.
    d. both a and c.

True or false

26. _____ The membranous labyrinth is filled with endolymph.

27. _____ The correct order of the auditory ossicles from deep to the tympanic membrane is incus, malleus, and stapes.

28. _____ If the hairs of the organ of Corti are damaged, nerve deafness results—even if the vestibulocochlear nerve is healthy.

29. _____ Movement of the tympanic membrane from sound waves initiates vibration of the auditory ossicles.

30. _____ *Vertigo* essentially means "fear of heights."

Labeling—identify the structures of the ear by matching each term with its corresponding number on the following illustration.

_____ auditory tube

_____ stapes

_____ cochlea

_____ semicircular canals

_____ facial nerve

_____ external auditory meatus

_____ malleus

_____ round window

_____ auricle

_____ vestibular nerve

_____ oval window

_____ incus

_____ vestibule

_____ temporal bone

_____ cochlear nerve

_____ tympanic membrane

(Not to scale)

▷ *If you had difficulty with this section, review pages 564-570.*

IV—VISION: THE EYE

Multiple Choice—select the best answer.

31. From superficial to deep, the three layers of tissue that compose the eyeball are:
    a. sclera, retina, choroid.
    b. choroid, sclera, retina.
    c. sclera, choroid, retina.
    d. retina, choroid, sclera.

32. The anterior portion of the sclera is called the:
    a. cornea.
    b. iris.
    c. lens.
    d. conjunctiva.

33. The neurons of the retina—in the order in which they conduct impulses—are:
    a. photoreceptor neurons, bipolar neurons, ganglion neurons.
    b. photoreceptor neurons, ganglion neurons, bipolar neurons.
    c. bipolar neurons, photoreceptor neurons, ganglion neurons.
    d. bipolar neurons, ganglion neurons, photoreceptor neurons.

34. All of the axons of ganglion neurons extend back to an area of the posterior eyeball called the:
    a. fovea centralis.
    b. macula lutea.
    c. canal of Schlemm.
    d. optic disc.

35. Which of the following spaces contains vitreous humor?
    a. anterior chamber
    b. posterior chamber
    c. anterior cavity
    d. posterior cavity

36. The white of the eye is called the:
    a. sclera.
    b. choroid.
    c. retina.
    d. cornea.

37. The function of the lacrimal gland is to:
    a. secrete aqueous humor.
    b. secrete vitreous humor.
    c. secrete tears.
    d. none of the above.

38. Accommodation of the lens for near vision necessitates:
    a. increased curvature of the lens.
    b. relaxation of the ciliary muscle.
    c. contraction of the suspensory ligament.
    d. dilation of the pupil.

39. People whose acuity is worse than 20/200 after correction are considered to be:
    a. nearsighted.
    b. farsighted.
    c. legally blind.
    d. none of the above.

40. An intrinsic eye muscle is the:
    a. iris.
    b. pupil.
    c. sclera.
    d. retina.

True or false

41. _____ The canal of Schlemm drains the vitreous humor from the anterior chamber.

42. _____ All the muscles associated with the eye are smooth or involuntary.

43. _____ Conjunctivitis is a highly contagious infection.

44. _____ The correct order of flow of tears is as follows: lacrimal gland, lacrimal duct, punctum, lacrimal canal, lacrimal sac, and nasolacrimal duct.

45. _____ Deficiency of the blue-sensitive photopigments is the most common form of color blindness.

46. _____ The opening and separation of opsin and retina in the presence of light is called *bleaching*.

47. _____   The retina is the incomplete in-nermost coat of the eyeball in that it has no anterior portion.

48. _____   *Refraction* means "the deflection or bending of light rays."

49. _____   A person with a 20/100 vision can see objects at 100 feet that a person with normal vision can see at 20 feet.

50. _____   A person with strabismus usually has double vision.

Labeling—label the horizontal section through the eyeball on the following illustration.

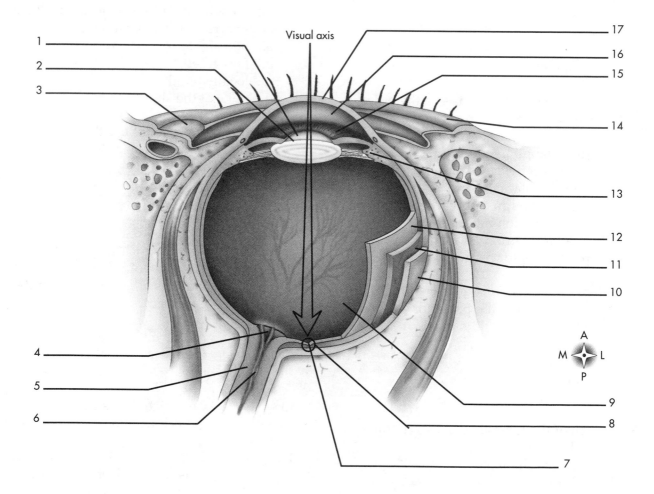

Labeling—label the extrinsic muscles of the right eye on the following illustration.

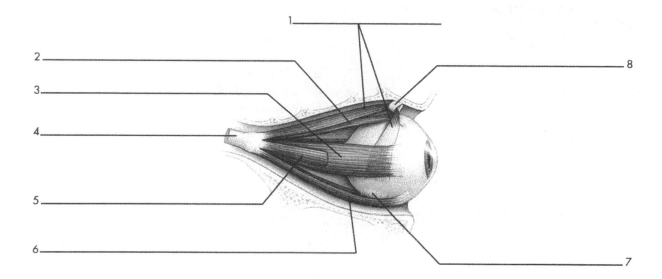

Labeling—label the structures of the lacrimal apparatus on the following illustration.

▷ *If you had difficulty with this section, review pages 571-580.*

V—MECHANISMS OF DISEASE

Matching—identify the best answer from the choices given and insert the letter in the answer blank.

a. tinnitus
b. presbycusis
c. otosclerosis
d. otitis media
e. vertigo
f. Ménière disease

51. _____ inherited bone disorder that impairs conduction by causing structural irregularities in the stapes

52. _____ "ringing in the ear"

53. _____ middle ear infection

54. _____ sensation of spinning

55. _____ progressive hearing loss associated with aging

56. _____ chronic inner ear disease characterized by progressive nerve deafness and vertigo

Matching—select the best answer from the choices given and insert the letter in the answer blank.

a. trachoma
b. retinopathy
c. myopia
d. glaucoma
e. astigmatism
f. conjunctivitis
g. nyctalopia
h. hyperopia
i. scotoma
j. cataracts

57. _____ nearsightedness

58. _____ an irregularity in the cornea

59. _____ "pink-eye"

60. _____ Chlamydial conjunctivitis

61. _____ cloudy spots in the eye's lens

62. _____ often caused by diabetes mellitus

63. _____ farsightedness

64. _____ "night blindness"

65. _____ loss of only the center of the visual field

66. _____ excessive intraocular pressure caused by abnormal accumulation of aqueous humor

▷ *If you had difficulty with this section, review pages 580-584.*

Crossword Puzzle

Across

1. Photopigment in rods
4. "Snail"
8. Provides information related to head position or acceleration
10. Smell

Down

2. Pain receptor
3. Deflection of light rays
5. Inner ear
6. Crista _____; dynamic equilibrium
7. Taste
9. Innermost coat of eyeball

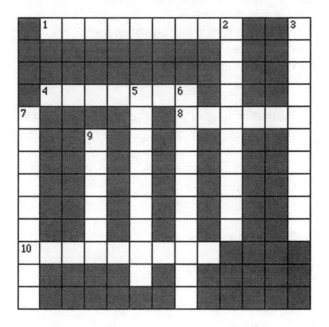

APPLYING WHAT YOU KNOW

67. Kim became ill repeatedly with throat infections during her first few years of school. Lately, however, she has noticed that when ever she has a throat infection, her ears become very sore also. What might be the cause of this additional problem?

68. Deb is a woman with unusually poor vision. Without glasses, she needs to stand 20 feet away from an object to see it, whereas a person with normal vision could see that same object from 400 feet. How would you quantify her visual acuity? What must she score in a visual acuity exam after correction with glasses to avoid being designated as legally blind? With which type of refraction disorder is she afflicted? What shape lenses would be required to focus a clear image on her retina?

DID YOU KNOW?

- Synesthesia is a rare condition in which the senses are combined. Synesthetes see words, taste colors and shapes, and feel flavors.

- A human can taste one gram of salt in 500 liters of water (0.0001M).

ONE LAST QUICK CHECK

Multiple Choice—select the best answer.

69. Where are the specialized mechanoreceptors of hearing and balance located?
    a. inner ear
    b. malleus
    c. helix
    d. all of the above

70. The organ of Corti is the sense organ of what sense?
    a. sight
    b. hearing
    c. pressure
    d. taste

71. Where are taste sensations interpreted?
    a. cerebral cortex
    b. nasal cavity
    c. area of stimulation
    d. none of the above

72. An eye physician is a/an:
    a. oculist.
    b. optometrist.
    c. ophthalmologist.
    d. none of the above.

73. Which of the following statements about the sclera is true?
    a. It is a mucous membrane.
    b. It is called the *white of the eye*.
    c. It lies behind the iris.
    d. All of the above are true.

74. Which of the following are encapsulated nerve endings?
    a. gustatory receptors
    b. pacinian corpuscles
    c. olfactory receptors
    d. all of the above

75. The retina contains microscopic receptor cells called:
    a. mechanoreceptors.
    b. chemoreceptors.
    c. olfactory receptors.
    d. rods and cones.

76. Which two involuntary muscles make up the front part of the eye?
    a. malleus and incus
    b. iris and ciliary muscle
    c. retina and pacinian muscle
    d. sclera and iris

77. Which of the following statements about gustatory sense organs is true?
    a. They are called *taste buds*.
    b. The are innervated by cranial nerves VII and IX.
    c. They work together with the olfactory senses.
    d. All of the above are true.

78. The external ear consists of the:
    a. auricle and auditory canal.
    b. labyrinth.
    c. organ of Corti and cochlea.
    d. none of the above.

True or false

79. _____ The tympanic membrane separates the middle ear from the external ear.

80. _____ Glaucoma may result from a blockage of flow of vitreous humor.

81. _____ With the condition of presbyopia the eye lens loses its elasticity.

82. _____ The crista ampullaris is located in the nasal cavity.

83. _____ Myopia occurs when images are focused in front of the retina rather than on it.

84. _____ Light enters through the pupil and the size of the pupil is regulated by the iris.

85. _____ The retina is the innermost layer of the eye and contains structures called *rods*.

86. _____ The olfactory receptors are chemical receptors.

87. _____ Meissner's corpuscle is a tactile corpuscle.

88. _____ The macula provides information related to head position or acceleration.

CHAPTER 16

Endocrine System

The endocrine system has often been compared to a fine concert symphony. When all instruments are playing properly, the sound is melodious. If one instrument plays too loud or too soft, however, it affects the overall quality of the entire performance.

The endocrine system is a ductless system that releases hormones into the bloodstream to help regulate body functions. The pituitary gland may be considered the conductor of the orchestra, because it stimulates many of the endocrine glands to secrete their powerful hormones. All hormones, whether stimulated in this manner or by other control mechanisms, are interdependent. A change in the level of one hormone may affect the level of many other hormones.

In addition to the endocrine glands, prostaglandins, or "tissue hormones," are powerful substances similar to hormones that have been found in a variety of body tissues. These hormones are often produced in a tissue and diffuse only a short distance to act on cells within that area. Prostaglandins influence respiration, blood pressure, gastrointestinal secretions, and the reproductive system and may some day play an important role in the treatment of diseases such as hypertension, asthma, and ulcers.

The endocrine system is a system of communication and control. It differs from the nervous system in that hormones provide a slower, longer-lasting effect than do nerve stimuli and responses. Your understanding of the "system of hormones" will alert you to the mechanism of our emotions, response to stress, growth, chemical balances, and many other body functions.

I—THE ENDOCRINE SYSTEM AND HORMONES

Multiple Choice—select the best answer.

1. The chemical messengers of the endocrine system are:
   a. hormones.
   b. neurotransmitters.
   c. target tissues.
   d. target organs.

2. Which of the following statements is true of the endocrine system?
   a. The cells secreting the chemical messengers are called *neurons*.
   b. The distance traveled by the chemical messengers is short (across a microscopic synapse).
   c. Its effects are slow to appear, yet long-lasting.
   d. None of the above. Hormone receptors are nonspecific

3. Which of the following is *NOT* an endocrine gland?
   a. pineal
   b. placenta ovaries
   c. parathyroid
   d. intestines

4. The neuroendocrine system performs all of the following *EXCEPT*:
   a. communication.
   b. control.
   c. conduction.
   d. integration.

5. The many hormones secreted by endocrine tissues can be classified simply as:
   a. steroid or nonsteroid hormones.
   b. anabolic or catabolic hormones.
   c. sex or nonsex hormones.
   d. tropic or hypotropic hormones.

6. Nonsteroid hormones include:
   a. proteins.
   b. peptides.
   c. glycoproteins.
   d. all of the above.

7. Anabolic hormones:
   a. target other endocrine glands and stimulate their growth and secretion.
   b. target reproductive tissue.
   c. stimulate anabolism in their target cells.
   d. stimulate catabolism in their target cells.

8. The second messenger most often involved in nonsteroid hormone action is:
   a. cAMP.
   b. mRNA.
   c. ATP.
   d. GTP.

9. The control of hormone secretion is:
   a. usually part of a negative feedback loop.
   b. rarely part of a positive feedback loop.
   c. both a and b.
   d. none of the above.

10. When a small amount of hormone allows a second hormone to have its full effect on a target cell, the phenomenon is called:
    a. synergism.
    b. permissiveness.
    c. antagonism.
    d. combination.

True or false

11. ___T___ The nervous system functions at a much greater speed than the endocrine system.

12. ___T___ The most widely used method of hormone classification is by chemical structure.

13. ___F___ Steroid hormone receptors are usually attached in the plasma membrane of a target cell.

14. ___F___ Production of too much hormone of a diseased gland is termed *hyposecretion*.

15. ___T___ Input from the nervous system influences secretions of hormones.

Labeling—label the location and structure of the pituitary gland on the following illustration.

▷ *If you had difficulty with this section, review pages 607-612.*

IV—PINEAL, THYROID, AND PARATHYROID GLANDS

Multiple Choice—select the best answer.

32. Which thyroid hormone is released in greatest quantity?
    a. T_3
    b. T_4
    c. triiodothyronine
    d. calcitonin

33. The principal thyroid hormone is:
    a. thyroxine.
    b. triiodothyronine.
    c. T_4.
    d. both a and c.

34. The two lobes of the thyroid are connected by the:
    a. infundibulum.
    b. isthmus.
    c. peninsula.
    d. islet.

35. High blood calcium levels can cause all of the following *EXCEPT*:
    a. constipation.
    b. muscle spasms.
    c. lethargy.
    d. coma.

36. PTH increases calcium absorption in the intestines by activating:
    a. vitamin A.
    b. vitamin C.
    c. vitamin D.
    d. iron.

True or false

37. _____ Calcitonin in humans does not seem to have a great effect.

38. _____ The parathyroid glands are located on the anterior surface of the thyroid gland.

39. _____ Hypersecretion of thyroid hormone can cause Graves disease.

40. _____ The pineal gland functions to support the body's biological clock.

41. _____ The structural units of thyroid tissue are called *colloids*.

Labeling—label the following illustration showing the structure of the thyroid and parathyroid glands.

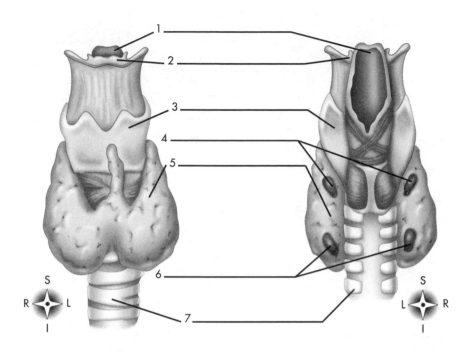

1 _____

2 _____

3 _____

4 _____

5 _____

6 _____

7 _____

S
R ✦ L
I

S
L ✦ R
I

▷ *If you had difficulty with this section, review pages 613-618.*

V—ADRENAL GLANDS

Multiple Choice—select the best answer.

42. Which of the following hormones is *NOT* secreted by the adrenal cortex?
    a. aldosterone
    b. epinephrine
    c. adrenal androgens
    d. adrenal estrogens

43. Which of the following hormones is *NOT* secreted by the adrenal medulla?
    a. epinephrine
    b. norepinephrine
    c. adrenaline
    d. all of the above are secreted by adrenal medulla

44. The most physiologically important miner-alocorticoid is:
    a. aldosterone.
    b. angiotensin II.
    c. renin.
    d. angiotensin I.

True or false

45. ____ T ____   The outer portion of an adrenal gland is called the *adrenal cortex*.

46. ____ F ____   Hypersecretion of cortisol from the adrenal cortex produces a collection of symptoms called *Addison disease*.

47. ____ T ____   The renin-angiotensin mechanism is a negative feedback mechanism that helps maintain homeostasis of blood pressure.

▷ *If you had difficulty with this section, review pages 619-625.*

VI—PANCREATIC ISLETS

Multiple Choice—select the best answer.

48. Glucagon functions to:
    a. promote the entry of glucose into cells.
    b. convert glucose into glycogen.
    c. increase blood glucose concentration.
    d. decrease blood glucose concentration.

49. Insulin functions to:
    a. decrease blood concentration of glucose, amino acids, and fatty acids.
    b. increase blood concentration of glucose, amino acids, and fatty acids.
    c. inhibit the secretion of growth hormone.
    d. both a and c.

True or false

50. _____ Somatostatin has the primary role of inhibiting the secretion of the other pancreatic hormone.

51. _____ Pancreatic polypeptide is the dominant pancreatic hormone in the regulation of blood glucose homeostasis.

Matching—identify each pancreatic islet cell type with its appropriate hormone secretion.

a. alpha cells
b. beta cells
c. delta cells
d. pancreatic polypeptide cells

52. _____ insulin

53. _____ somatostatin

54. _____ glucagon

55. _____ pancreatic polypeptide

▷ *If you had difficulty with this section, review pages 625-631.*

VII—OTHER ENDOCRINE GLANDS AND TISSUES

Multiple Choice—select the best answer.

56. The major hormone produced by the corpus luteum is:
    a. progesterone.
    b. estrogen.
    c. chorionic gonadotropin.
    d. none of the above.

57. Testosterone is produced by:
    a. seminiferous tubules.
    b. interstitial cells.
    c. LH.
    d. the scrotum.

58. The hormone that can be detected during the early part of a woman's pregnancy with an over-the-counter kit is:
    a. LH.
    b. estrogen.
    c. hCG.
    d. ANH.

True or false

59. _____ Thymosin is a major digestive hormone.

60. _____ Atrial natriuretic hormone aids in the homeostasis of blood volume and blood pressure.

61. _____ Secretin plays a major regulatory role in the digestive process.

▷ *If you had difficulty with this section, review pages 631-632.*

VIII—MECHANISMS OF DISEASE

Matching—identify the disease with its appropriate description.

a. hypersecretion of ACTH
b. lack of iodine
c. hypersecretion of thyroid hormone
d. hypersecretion of melatonin
e. hypersecretion of GH (adults)
f. extreme hyposecretion of thyroid (adult)
g. hyposecretion of estrogen in postmenopausal women
h. hyposecretion of adrenal cortex

62. _____ acromegaly

63. _____ Addison disease

64. _____ Cushing syndrome

65. _____ Graves disease

66. _____ myxedema

67. _____ osteoporosis

68. _____ simple goiter

69. _____ winter depression

▷ *If you had difficulty with this section, review pages 633-634.*

Crossword Puzzle

Across
2. Secretes thyroxin
3. Secretes parathormone
6. Secreted by endocrine system
7. Anterior pituitary
8. A cell with one or more receptors for a particular hormone (two words)
9. Posterior pituitary gland

Down
1. Located in the mediastinum beneath sternum
2. Hormones that target other endocrine glands (two words)
3. Tissue hormone
4. Secretes aldosterone
5. Primary sex organs

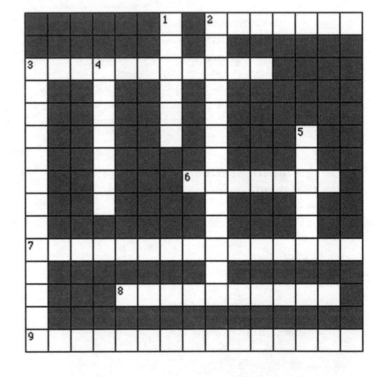

APPLYING WHAT YOU KNOW

70. After a visit with the doctor, Amanda and Bill were elated to learn of the high levels of human chorionic gonadotropin in Amanda's urine. Why would this couple be so delighted? Which organ produced this hormone in her body and what is its function?

71. Dania has been experiencing excessive thirst, hunger, and copious urination. Which endocrine system syndrome may she be experiencing? What are the actual physiological mechanisms that are causing her symptoms? How is she most likely to be treated?

Diabetes mellitus inadequate insulin or abnormal type of insulin, insulin injection.

72. India was pregnant and was 2 weeks past her due date. Her doctor suggested that she enter the hospital and he would induce labor. What hormone will he give India?

oxytocin

DID YOU KNOW

- People with dwarfism almost always have normal-sized children, even if both parents have dwarfism.

- The pituitary weighs little more than a small paper clip.

ONE LAST QUICK CHECK ✔

Multiple Choice—select the best answer.

73. What does the outer zone of the adrenal cortex secrete?
    a. mineralocorticoids
    b. sex hormones
    c. glucocorticoids
    d. epinephrine

74. From what condition does diabetes insipidus result?
    a. low insulin levels
    b. high glucagon levels
    c. low antidiuretic hormone levels
    d. high steroid levels

75. Which of the following statements is true regarding a young child whose growth is stunted, metabolism is low, sexual development is delayed, and mental development is retarded?
    a. The child may suffer from cretinism.
    b. The child may have an underactive thyroid.
    c. Profound manifestations of the described condition may result in deformed dwarfism.
    d. All of the above.

76. What can result when too much growth hormone is produced by the pituitary gland?
    a. hyperglycemia
    b. a pituitary giant
    c. both a and b
    d. none of the above

77. Which of the following glands is NOT regulated by the pituitary?
    a. thyroid
    b. ovaries
    c. adrenals
    d. thymus

78. Which of the following statements about the antidiuretic hormone is true?
    a. It is released by the posterior lobe of the pituitary.
    b. It causes diabetes insipidus when produced in insufficient amounts.
    c. It decreases urine volume.
    d. All of the above.

79. What controls the development of the body's immune system?
    a. pituitary
    b. thymus
    c. pineal body
    d. thyroid

80. Administration of which of the following would best treat a person suffering from rheumatoid arthritis?
    a. gonadocorticoids
    b. glucagon
    c. mineralocorticoids
    d. glucocorticoids

81. Which endocrine gland is composed of cell clusters called the *islets of Langerhans*?
    a. adrenals
    b. thyroid
    c. pituitary
    d. pancreas

82. Which of the following statements concerning prostaglandins is true?
    a. They control activities of widely separated organs.
    b. They can be called *tissue hormones*.
    c. They diffuse over long distances to act on cells.
    d. All of the above.

Asha is having difficulty breastfeeding and the lactating nurse su

Matching—select the most correct answer for each item (only one answer is correct).

a. glucocorticoid hormones
b. antidiuretic hormone
c. mineralocorticoid
d. oxytocin
e. growth hormone
f. placenta
g. luteinizing hormone
h. insulin
i. prolactin
j. thyroid hormones

83. _____ goiter

84. _____ ovulation

85. _____ diabetes mellitus

86. _____ lactation

87. _____ diabetes insipidus

88. _____ chorionic gonadotropins

89. _____ Cushing syndrome

90. _____ labor

91. _____ acromegaly

92. _____ aldosterone

CHAPTER 17

Blood

Blood, the river of life, is the body's primary means of transportation. Although it is the respiratory system that provides oxygen for the body, the digestive system that provides nutrients, and the urinary system that eliminates wastes, none of these functions could be provided for the individual cells without the blood. In less than one minute, a drop of blood will complete a trip through the entire body, distributing nutrients and collecting the wastes of metabolism.

Blood is divided into plasma (the liquid portion of blood) and the formed elements (the blood cells). There are three types of blood cells: red blood cells, white blood cells, and platelets. Together these cells and plasma provide a means of transportation that delivers the body's daily necessities.

Although all of us have red blood cells that are similar in shape, we have different blood types. Blood types are identified by the presence of certain antigens in the red blood cells. Every person's blood belongs to one of four main blood groups: Type A, B, AB, or O. Any one of the four groups or "types" may or may not have the Rh factor present in the red blood cells. If an individual has a specific antigen called the *Rh factor* present in his or her blood, the blood is Rh positive. If this factor is missing, the blood is Rh negative. Approximately 85% of the population have the Rh factor (Rh positive) while 15% do not have the Rh factor (Rh negative).

Your understanding of this chapter is necessary to prepare a proper foundation for the study of the circulatory system.

I—COMPOSITION OF BLOOD AND RED BLOOD CELLS

Multiple Choice—select the best answer.

1. The composition of blood is:
    a. 55% plasma, 45% formed elements.
    b. 45% plasma, 55% formed elements.
    c. 50% plasma, 50% formed elements.
    d. none of the above.

2. A hematocrit of 45% means that in every 100 ml of whole blood:
    a. there are 45 ml of red blood cells and 55 ml of plasma.
    b. there are 45 ml of plasma and 55 ml of red blood cells.
    c. 45% of the formed elements are red blood cells.
    d. plasma is 45% of the circulating whole blood.

3. Reduced red blood cell numbers cause:
    a. polycythemia.
    b. buffy coat.
    c. anemia.
    d. both a and c.

4. Which of the following formed elements carry oxygen?
    a. leukocytes
    b. erythrocytes
    c. thrombocytes
    d. monocytes

5. All formed elements arise from which stem cell?
    a. proerythroblast
    b. megakaryoblast
    c. lymphoblast
    d. hemocytoblast

True or false

6. ___T___   *Hematocrit* and *packed cell volume (PCV)* are synonymous terms.

7. ___F___   A reticulocyte count can indicate to a physician the rate of leukocyte formation.

8. ___T___   Oxygen deficiency increases RBC numbers by increasing the secretion of erythropoietin by the kidneys.

9. ___F___   The life span of circulating RBCs is about 10 to 12 days.

10. ___F___   Heme is broken down into iron and amino acids for use in the synthesis of new RBCs.

Labeling—label the different types of leukocytes on the following illustration.

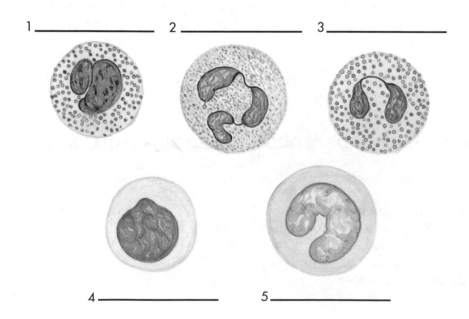

1 _____   2 _____   3 _____

4 _____   5 _____

▷ *If you had difficulty with this section, review pages 648-654.*

II—WHITE BLOOD CELLS AND PLATELETS

Matching—identify each term with its corresponding description.

a. agranulocytes
b. basophils
c. eosinophils
d. granulocytes
e. leukocytes
f. lymphocytes
g. megakaryocytes
h. monocytes
i. neutrophils
j. platelets

11. _____ classification of leukocytes that contain cytoplasmic granules

12. _____ most numerous leukocytes

13. _____ granulocytes that release heparin and histamine

14. _____ granulocytes that protect against infections from parasitic worms and allergic reactions

15. _____ agranulocytes that produce antibodies

16. _____ agranulocytes that enter tissue spaces as macrophages

17. _____ cell fragments that function in blood clotting and hemostasis

18. _____ cells from which platelets are formed

19. _____ classification of leukocytes without cytoplasmic granules

20. _____ classification of formed elements that are nucleated cells lacking hemoglobin

▶ *If you had difficulty with this section, review pages 655-658.*

III—BLOOD TYPES

Multiple Choice—select the best answer.

21. A person with antibody A in his or her plasma would have which blood type?
    a. type A
    b. type B
    c. type AB
    d. type O

22. People with type O blood are considered to be universal donors because their blood contains:
    a. neither A nor B antigens on their RBCs.
    b. both A and B antigens in their blood plasma.
    c. the Rh antigen on their RBCs.
    d. none of the above.

23. Blood transfusions are safer than ever due to:
    a. screening procedures such as the nucleic acid test.
    b. new freezing techniques.
    c. new phlebotomy techniques.
    d. all of the above.

True or false

24. ___T___ Type AB blood is considered to be the universal recipient.

25. ___F___ Type AB blood contains both the A and B antibodies in its plasma.

26. ___F___ Most blood contains the anti-Rh antibodies.

▶ *If you had difficulty with this section, review pages 658-662.*

IV—BLOOD PLASMA

True or false

27. _____ Plasma is a pale yellow fluid that accounts for more than half of the blood volume.

28. _____ Serum is whole blood minus the clotting elements.

29. _____   Synthesis of plasma proteins occurs in the spleen.

 If you had difficulty with this section, review page 662.

V—BLOOD CLOTTING

Multiple Choice—select the best answer.

30. Which of the following is *NOT* a critical component of coagulation?
    a. thrombin
    b. fibrinolysis
    c. fibrinogen
    d. fibrin

31. For prothrombin to be synthesized by the liver, adequate amounts of which vitamin is required?
    a. vitamin A
    b. vitamin C
    c. vitamin D
    d. vitamin K

32. Which of the following does *NOT* hasten clotting?
    a. rough spot in the endothelium
    b. abnormally slow blood flow
    c. heparin
    d. all of the above hasten clotting

If you had difficulty with this section, review pages 662-665.

VI—MECHANISMS OF DISEASE

Fill in the blanks.

33. _____ is an excess of RBCs.

34. _____ _____ often results from the destruction of bone marrow by drugs, toxic chemicals, or radiation.

35. An anemia resulting from a dietary deficiency of vitamin B_{12} is _____ _____.

36. A type of hemolytic anemia common to African-Americans is _____ _____ _____.

37. _____ refers to an abnormally low WBC count.

38. A _____ is a stationary clot.

39. A circulating clot is a(n) _____.

40. _____ is a type of X-linked inherited disorder that results from a failure to form blood-clotting factor VIII, IX, or XI.

If you had difficulty with this section, review pages 667-671.

Crossword Puzzle

Across

2. Liquid portion of blood
4. WBC
7. Thrombocyte
8. Blood cells (two words)
10. Least numerous of the WBCs
12. RBC formation
13. Oxygen-carrying mechanism of blood
14. Largest of the leukocytes

Down

1. Movement of formed elements through a vessel wall
3. Agglutinogen
5. RBC
6. 65% of WBCs
9. 2-5% of circulating WBCs
11. Agglutinin

APPLYING WHAT YOU KNOW

41. Pepper is an elite competitive cyclist who wanted to gain a physiological advantage over his competitors. He decided to have his own blood drawn and stored so that it could be infused into him prior to competition. What is the theory behind this practice? How effective is this procedure?

42. Mrs. Shearer's blood type is O positive. Her husband's type is O negative. Her newborn baby's blood type is O negative. Is there any need for concern with this combination?

43. After Mrs. Wiedeke's baby was born, the doctor applied a gauze dressing for a short time on the umbilical cord. He also gave the baby a dose of vitamin K. Why did the doctor perform these two procedures?

DID YOU KNOW

- In the second it takes to turn the page of a book, you will lose about 3 million red blood cells. During that same second, your bone marrow will have produced the same number of new ones.

- There is enough iron in a human to make a small nail.

ONE LAST QUICK CHECK

Multiple Choice—select the best answer.

44. Which of the following statements is false?
    a. Sickle cell anemia is caused by a genetic defect.
    b. Leukemia is characterized by a low number of WBCs.
    c. Polycythemia is characterized by an abnormally high number of erythrocytes.
    d. Pernicious anemia is caused by a lack of vitamin B_{12}.

45. Deficiency in the number or function of erythrocytes is called:
    a. leukemia.
    b. anemia.
    c. polycythemia.
    d. leukopenia.

46. Which of the following statements does *NOT* describe a characteristic of leukocytes?
    a. They are disc-shaped cells that do not contain a nucleus.
    b. They have the ability to fight infection.
    c. They provide defense against certain parasites.
    d. They provide immune defense.

47. Which of the following substances is *NOT* found in serum?
    a. clotting factors
    b. water
    c. hormones
    d. all of the above are found in serum

48. Which of the following substances is *NOT* found in blood plasma?
    a. water
    b. oxygen
    c. hormones
    d. none of the above

49. An allergic reaction may increase the number of:
    a. eosinophils.
    b. neutrophils.
    c. lymphocytes.
    d. monocytes.

50. What is a blood clot that is moving through the body called?
    a. embolism
    b. fibrosis
    c. heparin
    d. thrombosis

51. When could difficulty with the Rh blood factor arise?
    a. Rh-negative man and woman produce a child
    b. Rh-positive man and woman produce a child
    c. Rh-positive woman and an Rh-negative man produce a child
    d. Rh-negative woman and an Rh-positive man produce a child

52. What is the primary function of hemoglobin?
    a. fight infection
    b. produce blood clots
    c. carry oxygen
    d. transport hormones

53. Are any of the following steps *NOT* involved in blood clot formation?
    a. A blood vessel is injured and platelet factors are formed.
    b. Thrombin is converted into prothrombin.
    c. Fibrinogen is converted into fibrin.
    d. All of the above are involved in blood clot formation.

Matching—select the most correct answer for each item.

a. heparin
b. contains anti-A and anti-B antibodies
c. clotting
d. immunity
e. erythroblastosis fetalis
f. anemia
g. cancer
h. contains A and B antigens
i. reinfusion into self
j. phagocytosis
k. volume percent of RBCs in whole blood
l. decrease in WBCs

54. _____   lymphocytes

55. _____   erythrocyte disorder

56. _____   type AB

57. _____   basophils

58. _____   leukemia

59. _____   platelets

60. _____   type O

61. _____   Rh factor

62. _____   autologous transfusion

63. _____   neutrophils

64. _____   leukopenia

65. _____   hematocrit

CHAPTER 18

Anatomy of the Cardiovascular System

The heart is actually two pumps—one moves blood to the lungs, the other pushes it out into the body. These two functions seem rather elementary in comparison to the complex and numerous functions performed by most of the other body organs, and yet if this pump stops, within a few short minutes all life ceases.

The heart is divided into two upper compartments called *atria*, or receiving chambers, and two lower compartments, or discharging chambers, called *ventricles*. By age 45, approximately 300,000 tons of blood will have passed through these chambers to be circulated to the blood vessels. This closed system of circulation provides distribution of blood to the entire body (systemic circulation) and to specific regions, such as the pulmonary circulation or coronary circulation.

One hundred thousand miles of blood vessels make up the elaborate transportation system that circulates materials for energy, growth, and repair, and eliminates wastes from your body. These vessels are called *arteries, veins,* and *capillaries* (which are exchange vessels, or connecting links, between the arteries and veins). The pumping action of the heart keeps blood moving through the closed system of vessels. This closed system of circulation provides distribution of blood to the entire body and to specific regions such as the pulmonary circulation or hepatic portal circulation. Your review of the anatomy of this system will provide you with an understanding of the complex transportation mechanism necessary to provide oxygen and nutrients to our tissues.

I—HEART

Multiple Choice—select the best answer.

1. The visceral pericardium is found:
    a. inside the fibrous pericardium.
    b. adhering to the surface of the heart.
    c. lining the inside of the chambers of the heart.
    d. comprising the bulk of the heart tissue.

2. The correct layers of the heart, from superficial to deep, are:
    a. myocardium, pericardium, endocardium.
    b. epicardium, myocardium, pericardium.
    c. epicardium, myocardium, endocardium.
    d. endocardium, myocardium, epicardium.

3. The atrioventricular valves are also called:
    a. cuspid valves.
    b. semilunar valves.
    c. aortic valves.
    d. pulmonary valves.

4. Respectively, the right and left atrioventricular valves are also referred to as:
    a. tricuspid, mitral.
    b. bicuspid, tricuspid.
    c. mitral, bicuspid.
    d. bicuspid, mitral.

5. Semilunar valves prevent backflow of blood into the:
    a. atria.
    b. lungs.
    c. vena cava.
    d. ventricles.

6. The most abundant blood supply goes to the:
    a. right atrium.
    b. right ventricle.
    c. left atrium.
    d. left ventricle.

7. Branching of an artery as it progresses from proximal to distal is called:
    a. ischemia.
    b. infarction.
    c. anastomosis.
    d. both a and c.

8. The cavity of the heart that normally has the thickest wall is the:
    a. right atrium.
    b. right ventricle.
    c. left atrium.
    d. left ventricle.

9. Which of the following is a semilunar valve?
    a. aortic
    b. pulmonary
    c. mitral
    d. both a and b

10. The pacemaker of the heart is/are the:
    a. AV bundle.
    b. SA node.
    c. AV node.
    d. Purkinje fibers.

Labeling

11. Trace the blood flow through the heart by numbering the following structures in the correct sequence. Start with number 1 for the vena cava and proceed until you have numbered all the structures.

_____   tricuspid

_____   pulmonary veins

_____   pulmonary arteries

_____   pulmonary semilunar valve

_____   bicuspid valve

_____   left ventricle

_____   vena cava

_____   right atrium

_____   right ventricle

_____   left atrium

_____   aorta

_____   aortic semilunar valve

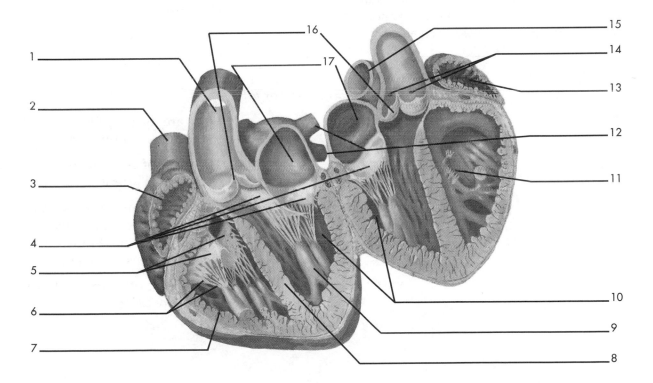

▷ *If you had difficulty with this section, review pages 678-687 and 690.*

Fill in the blanks.

12. A noninvasive technique for evaluating the internal structures and motions of the heart and great vessels is known as

_____.

13. Increased serum levels in the blood are often indicative of a recent myocardial infarction. These levels are monitored by blood tests known as _____

_____ _____.

14. A safe, noninvasive method of evaluating blood flow in coronary arteries or to evaluate ventricular function is

_____

_____

_____.

15. Rhythmic compressions of the heart combined with effective artificial respiration in cases of cardiac arrest is known as

_____

_____.

▷ *If you had difficulty with this section, review pages 678-691.*

II—BLOOD VESSELS

Matching—identify the term with the proper selection.

a. smooth muscle cells that guard the entrance to capillaries
b. carry blood to the heart
c. carry blood into the venules
d. carry blood away from the heart
e. outermost layers of arteries and veins
f. capillary that has a large lumen and more tortuous course than other capillary vessels
g. endothelium

16. _____ arteries

17. _____ capillaries

18. _____ tunica adventitia

19. _____ tunica intima

20. _____ sinusoid

21. _____ veins

22. _____ precapillary sphincters

True or false

23. _____ Veins are the only blood vessels to contain semilunar valves.

24. _____ The walls of veins are much thicker than arteries.

25. _____ Arteries become progressively smaller as blood flows away from the heart and into branches feeding other areas of the body.

26. _____ Arteries are often referred to as *capacitance vessels.*

Labeling—label the structure of blood vessels depicted in the following diagrams.

▷ *If you had difficulty with this section, review pages 692-695.*

III—MAJOR BLOOD VESSELS

Multiple Choice—select the best answer.

27. The aorta carries blood out of the:
   a. right atrium.
   b. right ventricle.
   c. left atrium.
   d. left ventricle.

28. The superior vena cava returns blood to the:
   a. left atrium.
   b. left ventricle.
   c. right atrium.
   d. right ventricle.

29. Blood returns from the lungs during pulmonary circulation via the:
   a. pulmonary artery.
   b. pulmonary veins.
   c. aorta.
   d. inferior vena cava.

30. The hepatic portal circulation serves the body by:
   a. removing excess glucose and storing it in the liver as glycogen.
   b. detoxifying blood.
   c. assisting the body to maintain proper blood glucose.
   d. all of the above.

31. The structure used to bypass the liver in the fetal circulation is the:
   a. foramen ovale.
   b. ductus venosus.
   c. ductus arteriosus.
   d. umbilical vein.

32. The foramen ovale serves the fetal circulation by:
    a. connecting the aorta and the pulmonary artery.
    b. shunting blood from the right atrium directly into the left atrium.
    c. bypassing the liver.
    d. bypassing the lungs.

33. The structure used to connect the aorta and pulmonary artery in the fetal circulation is the:
    a. ductus arteriosus.
    b. ductus venosus.
    c. aorta.
    d. foramen ovale.

34. Which of the following is *NOT* an artery?
    a. femoral
    b. popliteal
    c. coronary
    d. inferior vena cava

Fill in the blanks.

35. Blood flow from the heart to all parts of the body and back again is known as _____ _____.

36. Small vessels join the anterior and posterior arteries to form an arterial circle at the base of the brain known as the _____ _____ _____.

37. _____ are the ultimate extensions of capillaries.

38. When blood is in the capillaries of abdominal digestive organs, it must flow through the _____ _____ _____.

39. If either hepatic portal circulation or venous return from the liver is interfered with, a condition known as _____ may occur.

40. Two _____ _____ carry circulation to the placenta and one _____ _____ returns blood from the placenta.

41. Many arteries have corresponding _____ with the same name.

Labeling—label the principal veins of the body on the following illustration.

Labeling—label the principal arteries of the body on the following illustration.

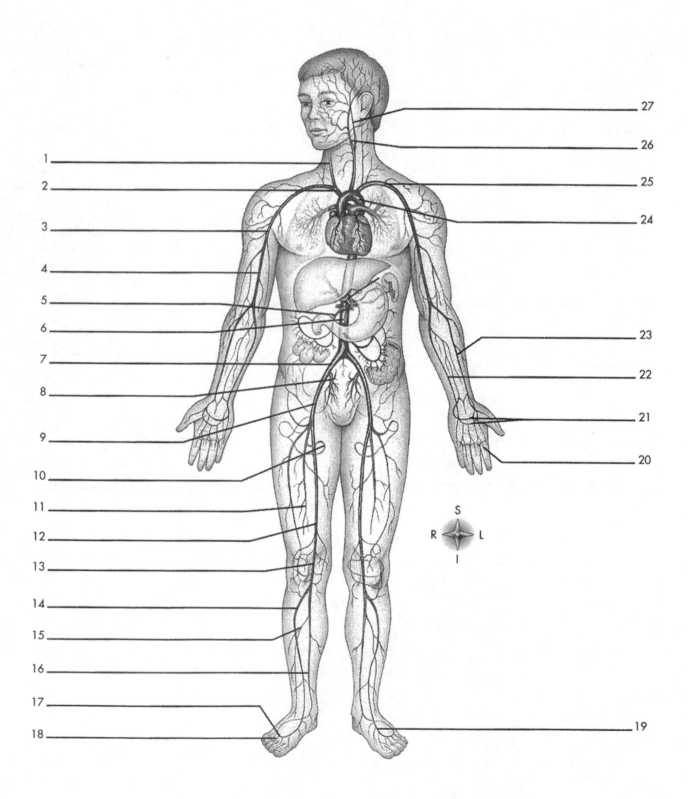

- Capillaries are so small that it takes ten of them to equal the thickness of a human hair.

- In one day, the blood travels a total of 12,000 miles... that's four times the distance across the U.S. from coast to coast!

ONE LAST QUICK CHECK ✔

Multiple Choice—select the best answer.

57. The superior vena cava carries blood to the:
    a. left ventricle.
    b. coronary arteries.
    c. right atrium.
    d. pulmonary veins.

58. Which of the following statements is *NOT* true regarding pericarditis?
    a. It may be caused by infection or trauma.
    b. It often causes severe chest pain.
    c. It may result in impairment of the pumping action of the heart.
    d. All of the above statements are true.

59. The outside covering that surrounds and protects the heart is called the:
    a. endocardium.
    b. myocardium.
    c. pericardium.
    d. ectocardium.

60. A valve that permits blood to flow from the right ventricle into the pulmonary artery is called the:
    a. tricuspid.
    b. mitral.
    c. aortic semilunar.
    d. pulmonary semilunar.

61. Hemorrhoids can best be described as:
    a. varicose veins.
    b. varicose veins in the rectum.
    c. thrombophlebitis of the rectum.
    d. clot formation in the rectum.

62. A common type of vascular disease that occludes arteries by lipids and other substances is:
    a. an aneurysm.
    b. atherosclerosis.
    c. varicose veins.
    d. thrombophlebitis.

Matching—select the most appropriate answer for each item (there is only one correct answer for each item).

a. ischemia
b. phlebitis
c. foramen ovale
d. aneurysm
e. vena cava
f. angioplasty
g. aorta
h. pulmonary
i. great saphenous vein
j. heart attack

63. _____   largest artery

64. _____   decreased blood supply

65. _____   leg vein

66. _____   fetal circulation

67. _____   arterial procedure

68. _____   vein inflammation

69. _____   lung circulation

70. _____   weakened artery

71. _____   large vein that returns venous blood to the heart

72. _____   myocardial infarction

CHAPTER 19

Physiology of the Cardiovascular System

The beating of the heart must be coordinated in a rhythmic manner if the heart is to pump effectively. That is achieved by electrical impulses that are stimulated by specialized structures embedded in the walls of the heart. The sinoatrial node, atrioventricular node, bundle of His, and Purkinje fibers combine efforts to produce the tiny electrical currents necessary to contract the heart. A healthy heart is necessary to pump blood throughout the body to nourish and oxygenate cells continuously. Any interruption or failure of this system may result in serious pathology.

Blood pressure is the force of blood in the vessels. This force is highest in the arteries and lowest in the veins. Normal blood pressure varies among individuals and depends upon the volume of blood in the arteries. The larger the volume of blood in the arteries, the more pressure is exerted on the walls of the arteries and the higher the arterial pressure. Conversely, the less blood in the arteries, the lower the blood pressure.

A functional cardiovascular system is vital for survival because without circulation, tissues would lack a supply of oxygen and nutrients. Waste products would begin to accumulate and could become toxic. Your review of this system will provide you with an understanding of the complex transportation mechanism of the body necessary for survival.

I—HEMODYNAMICS AND THE HEART AS A PUMP

1. Under resting conditions, the SA node fires at an intrinsic rhythmical rate of:
    a. 65 to 70 beats per minute.
    b. 70 to 75 beats per minute.
    c. 75 to 80 beats per minute.
    d. 80 to 85 beats per minute.

2. The normal pattern of impulse conduction through the heart is:
    a. AV node, SA node, AV bundle, Purkinje fibers.
    b. SA node, AV node, AV bundle, Purkinje fibers.
    c. AV bundle, AV node, SA node, Purkinje fibers.
    d. AV node, SA node, Purkinje fibers, AV bundle.

3. An ECG P wave represents:
    a. depolarization of the atria.
    b. repolarization of the atria.
    c. depolarization of the ventricles.
    d. repolarization of the ventricles.

4. Repolarization of the atria is:
    a. clearly depicted by the QRS complex.
    b. masked by the massive ventricular depolarization.
    c. masked by the massive ventricular repolarization.
    d. none of the above.

5. Contraction of the ventricles produces:
    a. the first heart sound (lub).
    b. the second heart sound (dupp).
    c. both of these.
    d. none of these.

True or false

6. __T__   The contraction phase of the cardiac cycle is referred to as *systole*.

7. __F__   *Tachycardia* refers to a heartbeat of fewer than 50 beats per minute.

8. __T__   The term *dysrhythmia* refers to abnormal heart sounds.

9. _____   PVC is an acronym for *premature ventricular contraction*.

10. _____   Isovolumetric ventricular contraction occurs between the start of ventricular systole and the opening of the semilunar valves.

Labeling—label the following ECG deflection waves.

If you had difficulty with this section, review pages 734-744 and 770.

II—CIRCULATION AND BLOOD PRESSURE

Multiple Choice—select the best answer.

11. Blood pressure at the venae cavae and right atrium is:
    a. 120 mm Hg.
    b. 100 mm Hg.
    c. 80 mm Hg.
    d. 0 mm Hg.

12. Starling's law of the heart states that:
    a. blood flows from areas of high pressure to areas of low pressure.
    b. the volume of blood ejected from the ventricle is constant.
    c. the more stretched the heart fibers are at the beginning of a contraction, the stronger is their contraction.
    d. average heart rate is 72 beats per minute.

13. Parasympathetic control of the heart involves the:
    a. glossopharyngeal nerve (cranial nerve IX).
    b. vagus nerve (cranial nerve X).
    c. carotid sinus.
    d. aortic sinus.

14. The vagus nerve is said to act as a(n) _____ on the heart.
    a. temperature monitor
    b. positive feedback loop
    c. ejection mechanism
    d. brake

15. Under normal conditions, blood viscosity changes:
    a. frequently.
    b. during hemorrhage only.
    c. under stress.
    d. very little.

16. A dominance of sympathetic impulses increases heart rate and stroke volume and constricts reservoir vessels in response to:
    a. decreased O_2, increased CO_2, and/or decreased pH.
    b. increased O_2, increased CO_2, and/or decreased pH.
    c. decreased O_2, decreased CO_2, and/or decreased pH.
    d. decreased O_2, increased CO_2, and/or increased pH.

17. The difference between systolic and diastolic pressure is called:
    a. bruit pressure.
    b. pulse pressure.
    c. laminar pressure.
    d. none of the above.

18. The popliteal pulse point is found:
    a. at the bend of the elbow.
    b. on the dorsum of the foot.
    c. behind the knee.
    d. behind the medial malleolus.

19. Peripheral resistance is primarily affected by:
    a. the length of myocardial fibers.
    b. blood viscosity and the diameter of arterioles.
    c. the capacity of the blood reservoirs.
    d. the elasticity of the heart.

20. At rest, most of the body's blood supply resides in the:
    a. pulmonary loop.
    b. systemic arteries and arterioles.
    c. capillaries.
    d. systemic veins and venules.

True or false

21. _____ Stroke volume is determined by multiplying cardiac output and heart rate.

22. _____ A slow and weakly beating heart tends to have a decreased cardiac output.

a) 23. _____ Starling's law operates in humans as a major regulator of stroke volume under ordinary conditions.

24. _____ Cardiac output can increase from 5 to 6 L/min during strenuous exercise.

a) 25. __F__ Skeletal muscle is of minor consequence in venous blood return to the heart.

b) 26. __T__ The fluid that leaves the capillaries at the arterial end is eventually recovered by the venous end of the capillary.

c) 27. __T__ Systolic blood pressure is the force with which the blood is pushing against the artery wall when the ventricles are contracting.

d) 28. __T__ Velocity of blood decreases as blood flows from the aorta toward the capillaries.

29. _____ The axillary artery is one of the six arteries identified to stop arterial bleeding.

30. __T__ Hypercapnia acts as a major stimulant to chemoreceptors.

▷ *If you had difficulty with this section, review pages 744-769.*

III—MECHANISMS OF DISEASE

Fill in the blanks.

31. Complications of septicemia may result in _____ _____ .

32. _____ _____ results from any type of heart failure.

33. An acute type of allergic reaction called _____ results in _____ _____ .

34. _____ _____ results from widespread dilation of blood vessels caused by an imbalance in autonomic stimulation of smooth muscles in vessel walls.

35. Hypovolemia means_____ _____ _____ .

36. A type of septic shock that results from staphylococcal infections that begin in the vagina of menstruating women and spread to the blood is _____ _____ .

▷ *If you had difficulty with this section, review pages 769-773.*

Which of the following statements about Blood Flow is Incorrect?
a) Skeletal muscle contraction does not affect venous blood return to the heart.
b) The fluid that leaves the capillaries at the arterial end is eventually recovered by the venous end of the capillary
c) see above
d)

Crossword Puzzle

Across

1. Sensitive to pressure
3. Complete heartbeat (two words)
7. Volume pumped per heartbeat (two words)
8. Heart contracting
9. Heart at rest
10. Determined by stroke volume and heart rate (two words)

Down

1. SA node
2. Amount of blood returned to the heart by veins
4. Reflex that functions in hypoxia or hypercapnia emergencies
5. Increase in diameter of blood vessel
6. Resistance that helps determine arterial blood pressure

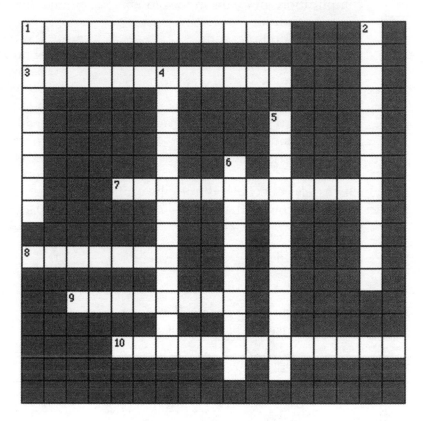

APPLYING WHAT YOU KNOW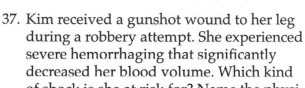

37. Kim received a gunshot wound to her leg during a robbery attempt. She experienced severe hemorrhaging that significantly decreased her blood volume. Which kind of shock is she at risk for? Name the physiological mechanisms that her body has initiated to attempt to maintain circulatory homeostasis.

38. Upon examination with electrocardiogram, Brian was diagnosed with a cardiac dysrhythmia that displayed very slow ventricular contractions and large intervals between the P wave and the R peak of the QRS complex. What is the physiological explanation for his symptoms? What can physicians do to restore his heart's conduction system?

DID YOU KNOW

what is the implication of there wit blood flow

- Every pound of excess fat contains 200 miles of additional capillaries. *440 km* *heart has to work harder to move blood.*

- If laid out in a straight line, the average adult's circulatory system would be nearly 60,000 miles long—enough to circle the earth 2.5 times.

ONE LAST QUICK CHECK

Multiple Choice—select the best answer.

39. The medical term for high blood pressure is:
    a. arteriosclerosis.
    b. cyanosis.
    c. hypertension.
    d. central venous pressure.

40. Septic shock is caused by:
    a. complications of toxins in the blood.
    b. a nerve condition.
    c. a drop in blood pressure.
    d. blood vessel dilation.

41. Hypovolemic shock is caused by:
    a. heart failure.
    b. dilated blood vessels.
    c. a drop in blood pressure.
    d. a severe allergic reaction.

42. Which vessels collect blood from the capillaries and return it to the heart?
    a. arteries
    b. sinuses
    c. veins
    d. arterioles

43. Which of the following events, if any, would NOT cause the blood pressure to increase?
    a. hemorrhaging
    b. increasing viscosity of the blood
    c. increasing the strength of the heartbeat
    d. all of the above

Matching—identify the most appropriate answer for each item.

a. P wave
b. abnormal heart rate
c. below 50 beats per minute
d. baroreflexes
e. hemodynamics
f. inadequate blood supply
g. diastole
h. excess carbon dioxide
i. residual volume
j. occur in carotid arteries
k. pacemaker
l. dorsalis pedis

44. _____ influences circulation of blood

45. _____ SA node

46. _____ depolarization of atria

47. _____ dysrhythmia

48. _____ bradycardia

49. _____ heart at rest

50. _____ blood remaining in ventricles

51. _____ pressoreflexes

52. _____ hypercapnia

53. _____ ischemia

54. _____ bruits

55. _____ pulse point

CHAPTER 20

Lymphatic System

The lymphatic system is similar to the circulatory system. Lymph, like blood, flows through an elaborate route of vessels. In addition to lymphatic vessels, the lymphatic system consists of lymph nodes, lymph, and the spleen. Unlike the circulatory system, the lymphatic vessels do not form a closed circuit. Lymph flows only once through the vessels before draining into the general blood circulation. This system is a filtering mechanism for microorganisms and serves as a protective device against foreign invaders, such as cancer.

As your text suggests, this system can also be likened to the wastewater system of our communities. Lymph circulates to bring contaminants to the system that are harmful to the body. Toxins are filtered and the fluid is returned cleansed, just as our wastewater systems remove harmful substances from the water and return it cleansed for our eventual use. Your knowledge of this system is necessary to understand the function of the lymphatic system in maintaining fluid balance in the tissues and the role that plays in the body's immune system.

I—LYMPHATIC VESSELS, LYMPH, AND CIRCULATION OF LYMPH

Multiple Choice—select the best answer.

1. The most important function(s) of the lymphatic system is/are:
   a. fluid balance of the internal environment.
   b. immunity.
   c. both a and b.
   d. none of the above.

2. Lymphatic capillaries that operate in the villi of the small intestine are called:
   a. lymphatics.
   b. lacteals.
   c. Peyer's patches.
   d. lymph nodes.

3. Lymph from the entire body drains into the thoracic duct, *EXCEPT* lymph from the:
   a. upper right quadrant.
   b. upper left quadrant.
   c. lower limbs.
   d. entire head and neck.

4. Which of the following is *NOT* a difference between lymphatics and veins?
   a. Lymphatics have thinner walls.
   b. Lymphatics contain more valves.
   c. Lymphatics contain lymph nodes.
   d. Lymphatics endure greater pressure.

5. If lymphatic return is blocked, which of the following will *NOT* occur?
   a. Blood protein concentration will fall.
   b. Blood osmotic pressure will fall.
   c. CO_2 levels in the blood will rise.
   d. Fluid imbalance will occur.

6. Lymphatic circulation is maintained by all of the following *EXCEPT*:
   a. breathing movements.
   b. heart.
   c. skeletal muscle contractions.
   d. valves.

7. Lymphatic circulation begins with lymphatic:
   a. capillaries.
   b. veins.
   c. venules.
   d. arterioles.

True or false

8. _____ The lymphatic system could be referred to as a specialized component of the circulatory system.

9. _____ Lymphatic vessels, like vessels in the blood vascular system, form a closed loop of circulation.

10. _____ Both lymph and interstitial fluid closely resemble blood plasma in composition.

11. _____ Lymph has a clotting ability similar to that of blood.

12. _____ The milky lymph found in lacteals after digestion is called *chyle*.

13. _____ A dilated structure on the thoracic duct that serves as a storage area for lymph moving toward its point of entry into the venous system is the cisterna chyli.

14. _____ Activities that result in central movement, or flow, of lymph are called *lymphokinetic actions*.

▶ *If you had difficulty with this section, review pages 780-785.*

II—LYMPH NODES

Multiple Choice—select the best answer.

15. The small depression of a lymph node from which the efferent lymph vessel arises is termed the:
    a. sinus.
    b. hilum.
    c. capsule.
    d. nodule.

16. The lymph nodes located in front of the ear are called the:
    a. submaxillary groups.
    b. inguinal lymph nodes.
    c. cervical lymph nodes.
    d. none of the above.

17. An infection of a lymph node is called:
    a. adenitis.
    b. noditis.
    c. lymphitis.
    d. lysis.

18. The lymphatic tissue of lymph nodes serves as the final maturation site for:
    a. monocytes.
    b. lymphocytes.
    c. both a and b.
    d. none of the above.

True or false

19. _____ Even though some lymph nodes occur in clusters, most occur as single nodes.

20. _____ Cortical nodules are composed of packed lymphocytes that surround an area called the *germinal center*.

Labeling—label the principal organs of the lymphatic system on the following illustration.

Labeling—label the structure of a lymph node on the following diagram.

▷ *If you had difficulty with this section, review pages 785-788.*

III—LYMPHATIC DRAINAGE OF THE BREAST

Multiple Choice—select the best answer.

21. Over 85% of the lymph from the breast enters lymph nodes of the:
    a. axillary region.
    b. supraclavicular region.
    c. brachial region.
    d. subscapular region.

22. The breast—mammary gland and surrounding tissue—is drained by:
    a. lymphatics that originate in and drain the skin over the breast, with exception of the areola and nipple.
    b. lymphatics that originate in and drain the substance of the breast itself, including the skin of the areola and nipple.
    c. both a and b.
    d. none of the above.

Labeling—label the lymphatic drainage of the breast on the following illustration.

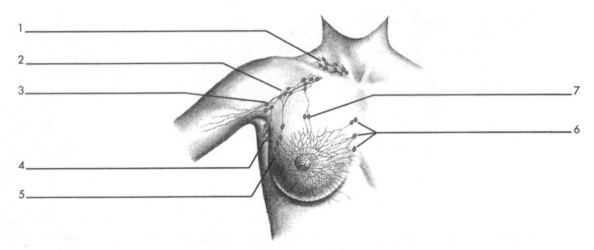

▷ *If you had difficulty with this section, review pages 788-789.*

IV—TONSILS, THYMUS, AND SPLEEN

Multiple Choice—select the best answer.

23. Adenoids are swollen:
    a. pharyngeal tonsils.
    b. palatine tonsils.
    c. lingual tonsils.
    d. none of the above.

24. The thymus secretes:
    a. T_3.
    b. T_4.
    c. thymosin.
    d. both a and c.

25. The thymus is located:
    a. deep to the thyroid.
    b. in the axillary region.
    c. in the mediastinum.
    d. none of the above.

True or false

26. ___F___ As a person ages, the thymus increases in size; this process is called *involution*.

27. _____ The spleen functions solely in the defense from foreign microorganisms.

28. ___T___ The spleen removes imperfect platelets from the blood.

▷ *If you had difficulty with this section, review pages 790-793.*

V—MECHANISMS OF DISEASE

Fill in the blanks.

29. _____ is a term that refers to a tumor of the cells of lymphoid tissue.

30. A middle ear infection is known as _____ _____ _____.

31. Septicemia is also known as _____ _____.

32. Lymphedema may be caused by small parasitic worms called _____ that infest the lymph nodes.

33. Two principal categories of lymphomas are _____ and _____ lymphoma.

▷ *If you had difficulty with this section, review pages 794-795.*

Crossword Puzzle

Across
4. Vessels that originate as lacteals in villi
5. Found in lacteals after digestion
6. Functions in defense and hematopoiesis (two words)
7. Palatine are an example
9. Active in production of T cells

Down
1. Activities that result in lymph flow
2. Destroys red blood cells
3. Located in villi
8. Fluid found in lymphatic vessels

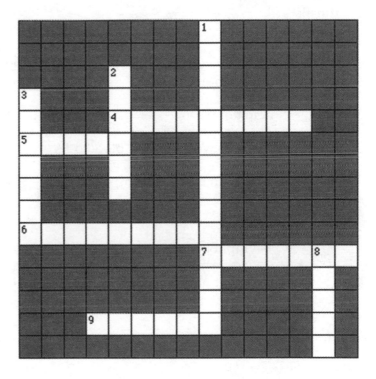

APPLYING WHAT YOU KNOW

34. Nancy was diagnosed with hemolytic anemia. Is a splenectomy a viable option? Can she live without her spleen? Why is removal of the spleen considered a treatment of choice?

35. Baby Wilson was born without a thymus gland. Immediate plans were made for a transplant to be performed. In the meantime, baby Wilson was placed in strict isolation. For what reason was he placed in isolation?

DID YOU KNOW ?

- According to the Centers for Disease Control and Prevention, 18 million courses of antibiotics are prescribed for the common cold in the United States per year. Research shows that colds are caused by viruses. Fifty million unnecessary antibiotics are prescribed for viral respiratory infections.

ONE LAST QUICK CHECK ✓

Matching—select the best response.

a. thymus
b. tonsils
c. spleen

36. _____ palatine, pharyngeal, and lingual are examples

37. _____ hematopoiesis

38. _____ destroys worn-out red blood cells

39. _____ located in mediastinum

40. _____ serves as a reservoir for blood

41. _____ T-lymphocytes

42. _____ largest at puberty

True or false

43. _____ The cisterna chyli is a dilated structure on the thoracic duct that serves as a storage area for lymph moving into the venous system.

44. _____ Healthy capillaries "leak" proteins.

45. _____ Thoracic duct lymph is "pumped" into the venous system during inspiration.

46. _____ Lymph nodes have several afferent and efferent vessels.

47. _____ Lymphedema is swelling due to an accumulation of lymph.

48. _____ An anastomosis is the removal of a part.

49. _____ The spleen is located below the diaphragm, above the right kidney and descending colon.

50. _____ Splenomegaly is removal of the spleen.

CHAPTER 21

Immune System

The immune system is the armed forces division of the body. Ready to attack at a moment's notice, the immune system defends us against the major enemies of the body: microorganisms, foreign transplanted tissue cells, and our own cells that have turned malignant.

The most numerous cells of the immune system are the lymphocytes. These cells circulate in the body's fluids seeking invading organisms and destroying them with powerful lymphotoxins, lymphokines, or antibodies.

Phagocytes, another large group of immune system cells, assist with the destruction of foreign invaders by a process known as *phagocytosis.* Neutrophils and macrophages ingest and digest the invaders, rendering them harmless to the body.

Another weapon that the immune system possesses is complement. Normally a group of inactive enzymes present in the blood, complement can be activated to kill invading cells by drilling holes in their cytoplasmic membranes, which allows fluid to enter the cell until it bursts. Your review of this chapter will give you an understanding of how the body defends itself from the daily invasion of destructive substances.

I—INNATE IMMUNITY

Multiple Choice—select the best answer.

1. Which of the following cells is *NOT* involved with innate immunity?
   a. natural killer cells
   b. neutrophils
   c. macrophages
   d. all of the above are involved with innate immunity

2. The "first line of defense" in innate immunity is:
   a. inflammation.
   b. phagocytosis.
   c. mechanical and chemical barriers.
   d. complement.

3. About 15% of the total number of lymphocyte cells are:
   a. natural killer (NK) cells.
   b. macrophages.
   c. neutrophils.
   d. interferon.

4. The most numerous type of phagocyte is the:
   a. neutrophil.
   b. macrophage.
   c. histocyte.
   d. Kupffer cell.

5. Which of the following is a phagocytic monocyte that migrates out of the bloodstream?
   a. neutrophil
   b. macrophage
   c. phagosome
   d. none of the above

True or false

6. ___F___ The immune mechanism that provides a general defense by acting against anything recognized as nonself is termed *adaptive immunity.*

7. _____ Species resistance is the genetic characteristics of the human species that protect the body from certain pathogens.

8. _____ Interferon has been proven effective as a treatment against most cancers.

9. _____ The complement cascade causes phagocytosis of the foreign cell that triggered it.

10. _____ Natural killer cells are a group of lymphocytes that kill many types of tumor cells and cells infected by different kinds of viruses.

▷ *If you had difficulty with this section, review pages 802-810.*

II—ADAPTIVE IMMUNITY

Multiple Choice—select the best answer.

11. B cells and T cells are examples of:
    a. monocytes.
    b. lymphocytes.
    c. neutrophils.
    d. macrophages.

12. Cell-mediated immunity involves:
    a. B cells.
    b. T cells.
    c. both a and b.
    d. neither a nor b.

13. The T cell subsets that are clinically important in diagnosing AIDS are:
    a. CD4.
    b. CD8.
    c. neither a nor b.
    d. both a and b.

14. An antibody consists of:
    a. two heavy and two light polypeptide chains.
    b. two heavy and one light polypeptide chains.
    c. one heavy and two light polypeptide chains.
    d. one heavy and one light polypeptide chains.

15. The amount of antibodies in a person's blood in response to exposure to a pathogen is called:
    a. toxoid.
    b. titer.
    c. both a and b.
    d. none of the above.

16. The most abundant circulating antibody is:
    a. IgM.
    b. IgG.
    c. IgA.
    d. IgE.

17. The specific cells that secrete antibodies are:
    a. B cells.
    b. T cells.
    c. plasma cells.
    d. none of the above.

18. T cells are sensitized by:
    a. direct exposure to an antigen.
    b. presentation of an antigen by a macro-phage.
    c. antibodies produced by B cells.
    d. lymphokines.

19. *Complement* can best be described as:
    a. an antibody.
    b. an enzyme in the blood plasma.
    c. a hormone.
    d. a lymphokine.

20. The chemical messengers that T cells release into inflamed tissues are called:
    a. pathogens.
    b. lymphokines.
    c. lymphotoxins.
    d. suppressor cells.

True or false

21. _____ Antibodies are proteins of the family called immunoglobulins.

22. _____ IgD is the most understood anti-body.

23. _____ The first vaccination was against the cowpox virus.

24. _____ Toxoids and vaccines function similarly.

25. _____ Active immunity generally lasts longer than passive immunity.

26. _____ Abnormal antigens or "tumor markers" are present in the plasma membranes of some cancer cells in addition to self-antigens.

27. _____ PSA is elevated in both benign and malignant prostate disease.

28. _____ Helper T cells and suppressor T cells help regulate adaptive immune function by regulating B cell and T cell function.

29. _____ A fetus receives protection from the mother through active artificial immunity.

30. _____ A vaccination provides natural passive immunity.

▷ *If you had difficulty with this section, review pages 811-830.*

III—MECHANISMS OF DISEASE

True or false

31. _____ The human immunodeficiency virus has a profound impact on a person's number of CD12 subset of T cells.

32. _____ Once inside a cell, HIV uses its viral RNA to produce DNA; this process is called *reverse transcription*.

33. _____ A common autoimmune disease is SLE or "lupus."

34. _____ SCID is an immunosuppressive drug.

35. _____ Glomerulonephritis is an autoimmune disease of the neuromuscular junction.

▷ *If you had difficulty with this section, review pages 829-834.*

Crossword Puzzle

Across

3. Family of cells descended from one cell
5. Cell-mediated immunity (two words)
7. Immunity that recognizes specific threatening agents and responds to these only
8. Inhibits spread of a viral infection
9. Enlarged monocytes that are giant phagocytic cells

Down

1. Produce antibodies (two words)
2. Immunity that resists various threatening agents (general defense)
4. Foreign protein
6. Plasma protein (immunoglobulin)

APPLYING WHAT YOU KNOW

36. Trent, a newborn, received immune protection from his mother through the placenta and breast milk. Which specific type of immunity is this? His older sister, Carrie, also recently received immune protection from a host of illnesses; however, hers was achieved deliberately via immunization by her pediatrician. What specific types of immunity is she experiencing? How do her types of immunity differ from her brother's?

37. Marcia is an intravenous drug user. She has developed a type of skin cancer known as Kaposi sarcoma. What, most likely, is Marcia's primary diagnosis? What are some of the medications that might be used to inhibit symptoms for a while?

DID YOU KNOW

- The swine flu vaccine in 1976 caused more deaths and illness than the disease that it was intended to prevent.

- In the United States, the HIV infection rate is increasing four times faster in women than in men. Women tend to underestimate their risk.

ONE LAST QUICK CHECK

Multiple Choice—select the best answer.

38. T cells do which of the following?
    a. develop in the thymus
    b. form memory cells
    c. form plasma cells
    d. all of the above

39. Acquired immune deficiency syndrome is characterized by which of the following?
    a. caused by a retrovirus
    b. causes inadequate T cell formation
    c. can result in death from cancer
    d. all of the above

40. Interferon is:
    a. produced by B cells.
    b. a protein compound that protects other cells by interfering with the ability of a virus to reproduce.
    c. a group of inactive enzyme proteins normally present in blood.
    d. all of the above.

41. B cells do which of the following?
    a. develop into plasma cells and memory cells
    b. secrete antibodies
    c. develop from primitive cells in bone marrow called *stem cells*
    d. all of the above

42. Which of the following functions to kill invading cells by drilling a hole in their plasma membrane?
    a. interferon
    b. complement
    c. antibody
    d. memory cell

43. What is a rapidly growing population of identical cells that produce large quantities of specific antibodies called?
    a. complementary
    b. lymphotoxic
    c. chemotactic
    d. monoclonal

44. Which of the following is a form of passive natural immunity?
    a. A child develops measles and acquires immunity to subsequent exposure.
    b. Antibodies are injected into an infected individual.
    c. An infant receives protection through its mother's milk.
    d. Vaccinations are given against small-pox.

Matching—identify the term with the proper selection.

a. inborn immunity
b. natural immunity
c. adaptive immunity
d. artificial exposure

45. _____ specific immunity

46. _____ inherited immunity

47. _____ acquired immunity

48. _____ immunization

CHAPTER 22

Stress

Life without any stress would be very dull and boring. Often it is stress that stimulates us to achieve our dreams and experience success and happiness. However, too much stress becomes unpleasant and tiring and can seriously interfere with our ability to function effectively. The challenge is to keep stress at a level that is healthy and enjoyable.

Although we react differently and in various degrees to stressors, we must acknowledge that in most individuals, stress leads to a physiological stress response. These responses may be as simple as an increase in heart rate or perspiration or as complex as a disease syndrome. And although we may not be aware of it on a day-to-day basis, stress can be cumulative and manifest itself long after apparent stressors have been resolved. Your study of this unit will alert you to the impact of stress on your body and the significant role it plays in homeostasis.

I—SELYE'S CONCEPT OF STRESS

Multiple Choice—select the best answer.

1. The stages of general adaptation syndrome in the correct order are:
   a. alarm reaction, stage of exhaustion, stage of resistance.
   b. alarm reaction, stage of resistance, stage of exhaustion.
   c. stage of exhaustion, alarm reaction, stage of resistance.
   d. stage of exhaustion, stage of resistance, stage of alarm.

2. The "stress triad" refers to:
   a. alarm, exhaustion, resistance.
   b. hypertrophied adrenals, atrophied thymus and lymph nodes, and bleeding ulcers.
   c. stressor, stress, and response.
   d. health, stress, and disease.

3. Which of the following is *NOT* an alarm reaction response resulting from hypertrophy of the adrenal cortex?
   a. hyperglycemia
   b. hypertrophy of thymus
   c. decreased immunity
   d. decreased allergic responses

4. All of the following are true statements *EXCEPT*:
   a. stressors are extreme stimuli.
   b. stressors are always unpleasant, injurious, or painful.
   c. the emotions of fear, anxiety, and grief can act as stressors.
   d. stressors differ in individuals.

5. What determines which stimuli are stressors for each individual?
   a. past experience
   b. diet
   c. heredity
   d. all of the above

True or false

6. _____ Selye's stage of exhaustion is reached in each exposure to stressors.

7. _____ High-stress, hard-driving, competitive individuals who may be at greater risk of coronary heart disease are classified as "Type B."

8. _____ The *stage of resistance* can also be described as *adaptation*.

9. _____ Stressors are "bad" stimuli that should always be avoided.

10. _____ The stress response commonly referred to as "fight or flight" is evoked by increased sympathetic activity.

▷ *If you had difficulty with this section, review pages 840-846.*

II—SOME CURRENT CONCEPTS ABOUT STRESS

Multiple Choice—select the best answer.

11. Corticotropin-releasing hormone (CRH) stimulates the anterior pituitary gland to secrete increased amounts of:
    a. glucocorticoids.
    b. aldosterone.
    c. ACTH.
    d. ADH.

12. All of the following are effects of cortisol *EXCEPT*:
    a. increased protein catabolism.
    b. decreased immune responses.
    c. decreased allergic responses.
    d. fight or flight responses.

13. The dominant subjective reaction that occurs with psychological stress is:
    a. guilt.
    b. anxiety.
    c. depression.
    d. fear.

True or false

14. _____ The current definition of *stress* is "any stimulus that directly or indirectly stimulates neurons of the hypothalamus to release corticotropin-releasing hormone (CRH)."

15. _____ It is accepted among physiologists that a higher-than-normal blood level of corticoids results in a greater ability to resist stress.

16. _____ Physiological stress and psychological stress are clearly different phenomena.

17. _____ Hypervolemia and antidiuresis are common responses to stress.

18. _____ Stress is an issue only among adolescents and adults.

▷ *If you had difficulty with this section, review pages 845-849.*

Crossword Puzzle

Across

1. General adaptation syndrome (abbrev.)
6. Agents that produce stress
7. Coping successfully with stress
8. General adaptation syndrome stage that develops only when stress is severe

Down

2. Also known as the stress response (two words)
3. Stage of general adaptation syndrome (two words)
4. General adaptation syndrome stage where sympathetic activity returns to normal
5. Hormones that increase during stress

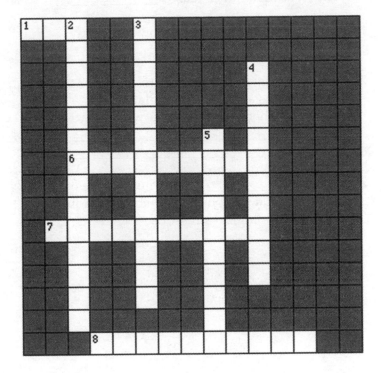

APPLYING WHAT YOU KNOW

19. Merrilee has an adolescent crush on John. Whenever she is near him, she feels anxious, her pupils dilate, heart rate elevates, systolic blood pressure rises, blood glucose levels are above normal, and blood and urine levels of epinephrine and norepinephrine are elevated. What is the physiological term used to describe this syndrome? Beginning in the hypothalamus, trace the mechanisms that are causing this response. If this physiological scenario were extended and intense, what illnesses might Merrilee be at risk for?

20. Bill is going to his boss for his annual evaluation. He is planning to ask for a raise and hopes the evaluation will be good. Which subdivision of the autonomic nervous system will be active during this stressful conference? Should he have a large meal before his appointment? Support your answer with facts.

DID YOU KNOW

• Laughing lowers levels of stress hormones and strengthens the immune system. Six-year-olds laugh an average of 300 times a day. Adults only laugh 15–100 times a day.

• A survey conducted at Iowa State College in 1969 suggests that a parent's stress at the time of conception plays a major role in determining a baby's sex. The child tends to be of the same sex as the parent who is under less stress.

ONE LAST QUICK CHECK

Fill in the blanks.

21. _____ _____ _____ is the term for the group of changes that make the presence of stress in the body known.

22. The stage of _____ develops only when stress is extremely severe or continues over a long period.

23. The hypothalamus releases _____

    _____ _____
    which acts as a trigger that initiates many
    diverse changes in the body.

24. The term that describes the stress responses
    that occur as a result of stimulation of
    the sympathetic centers is known as the

    _____ _____

    _____ _____.

25. _____ investigates
    physiological responses made by individu-
    als to psychological stressors.

True or False

26. _____   Type B personalities are at greater
             risk of coronary disease than
             Type A personalities.

27. _____   Stress causes disruption in ho-
             meostasis.

28. _____   Smoking increases plasma adre-
             nocorticoids by as much as 77%.

29. _____   Identical psychological stressors
             induce identical physiological re-
             sponses in different individuals.

30. _____   Hans Selye identified a group
             of changes classic to stress and
             called them the *stress triad*.

CHAPTER 23

Anatomy of the Respiratory System

As you sit reviewing this system your body needs 16 quarts of air per minute. Walking requires 24 quarts of air and running requires 50 quarts per minute. The respiratory system provides the air necessary for you to perform your daily activities and eliminates the waste gases from the air that you breathe. Take a deep breath and think of the air as entering some 250 million tiny air sacs similar in appearance to clusters of grapes. These microscopic air sacs expand to let air in and contract to force it out. These tiny sacs, or *alveoli*, are the functioning units of the respiratory system. They provide the necessary volume of oxygen and eliminate carbon dioxide 24 hours a day.

Air enters either through the mouth or the nasal cavity. Next it passes through the pharynx and past the epiglottis, through the glottis and the rest of the larynx. It then continues down the trachea, into the bronchi to the bronchioles, and finally through the alveoli. The reverse occurs for expelled air. Your review of this system is necessary to provide you with an understanding of this essential homeostatic mechanism—the breath of life.

I—UPPER RESPIRATORY TRACT

Multiple Choice—select the best answer.

1. Which of the following structures is *NOT* part of the upper respiratory tract?
   a. trachea
   b. larynx
   c. oropharynx
   d. nose

2. Which part of the respiratory system does *NOT* function as an air distributor?
   a. trachea
   b. bronchioles
   c. alveoli
   d. bronchi

3. Which sequence is the correct pathway for air movement through the nose and into the pharynx?
   a. anterior nares, posterior nares, vestibule, nasal cavity meati
   b. anterior nares, vestibule, posterior nares, nasal cavity meati
   c. nasal cavity meati, anterior nares, vestibule, posterior nares
   d. anterior nares, vestibule, nasal cavity meati, posterior nares

201

4. Which of the following is *NOT* a paranasal sinus?
   a. frontal
   b. maxillary
   c. mandibular
   d. sphenoid

5. The true vocal cords and the rima glottis are called the:
   a. glottis.
   b. epiglottis.
   c. vestibular fold.
   d. both a and b.

True or false

6. _____ Failure of the palatine bones to unite is called *cribriform palate.*

7. _____ The pharynx is a tubelike structure that opens only into the mouth and larynx.

8. _____ Enlarged pharyngeal tonsils are called *adenoids.*

9. _____ The more common name for the thyroid cartilage is *voicebox.*

10. _____ The epiglottis moves up and down during swallowing to prevent food or liquids from entering the trachea.

Labeling—using the terms provided, label the following illustration of the respiratory system.

bronchioles	larynx	laryngopharynx
upper respiratory tract	primary bronchi	lower respiratory tract
nasopharynx	oropharynx	alveolar sac
nasal cavity	trachea	alveolar duct

Labeling—label the structures of the nasal cavity on the following illustration.

1. _____
2. _____
3. _____
4. _____
5. _____
6. _____
7. _____

11. _____
10. _____
9. _____
8. _____

Labeling—using the terms provided, label the three divisions of the pharynx and nearby structures on the following illustration.

opening of the eustachian
  tube
laryngopharynx
esophagus
oropharynx

vocal cords
pharyngeal tonsil
epiglottis
uvula
lingual tonsil

hyoid bone
trachea
nasopharynx
soft palate
palatine tonsil

1. _____
2. _____
3. _____
4. _____
5. _____
6. _____

14. _____
13. _____
12. _____
11. _____
10. _____
9. _____
8. _____
7. _____

Labeling—label the structures related to the paranasal sinuses on the following illustration.

▷ *If you had difficulty with this section, review pages 856-861.*

II—LOWER RESPIRATORY TRACT

Multiple Choice—select the best answer.

11. Aspirated objects tend to lodge in the:
    a. right bronchus.
    b. left bronchus.
    c. either right or left bronchus.
    d. none of the above.

12. The fluid coating the alveoli that reduces surface tension is called:
    a. bronchus.
    b. surfactant.
    c. alveolus.
    d. none of the above.

13. Which of the following is *NOT* a subdivision of the thoracic cavity?
    a. left pleural division
    b. right pleural division
    c. medial pleural division
    d. mediastinum

14. Which of the following is *NOT* a true statement?
    a. When the diaphragm relaxes, it returns to a domelike shape.
    b. When the diaphragm contracts, it pulls the floor of the thoracic cavity downward.
    c. Changes in thorax size bring about inspiration and expiration.
    d. Raising the ribs decreases the depth and width of the thorax.

True or false

15. _____ The rings of cartilage that form the trachea are complete rings that prevent it from collapsing and shutting off the vital airway.

16. _____ The trachea divides into symmetrical primary bronchi.

17. _____ A tube is often placed in the tra-chea before a patient leaves the operating room, especially if he or she has had a muscle relaxant.

18. _____ The left lung is divided into three lobes by horizontal and oblique fissures.

19. _____ The apex of each lung is lateral and inferior.

20. _____ The exchange of gases between air and blood occurs in the al-veoli.

Labeling—label the lobes and fissures of the lungs on the following illustration (anterior view).

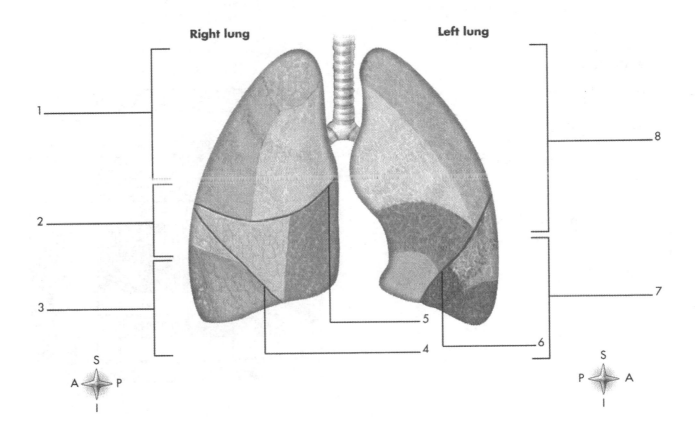

If you had difficulty with this section, review pages 862-872.

III—MECHANISMS OF DISEASE

Matching—identify each disorder with its corresponding description.

a. acute bronchitis
b. deviated septum
c. epistaxis
d. lung cancer
e. pharyngitis
f. rhinitis
g. tuberculosis
h. croup

21. _____ malignancy of pulmonary tissue

22. _____ very serious, chronic, and highly infectious infection

23. _____ displacement of the nasal septum

24. _____ a common infection of the lower respiratory tract characterized by acute inflammation of the bronchial tree

25. _____ nosebleed

26. _____ an inflammation of the mucosa of the nasal cavity

27. _____ sore throat

28. _____ harsh, vibrating cough

▷ *If you had difficulty with this section, review pages 872-878.*

Crossword Puzzle

Across

3. "Gas exchanger"
7. Trachea, two primary bronchi, and their branches (two words)
8. There are four pairs of these sinuses
9. Small branch of bronchus

Down

1. Serous membrane in the thoracic cavity
2. "Windpipe"
4. "Voice box"
5. "Throat"
6. Conchae

APPLYING WHAT YOU KNOW

29. Mrs. Metheny's 6-year-old child had trouble swallowing. She had a high fever, appeared very anxious, and was drooling from her mouth. Mrs. Metheny called the EMS personnel who assessed the child, inserted an airway, and transported her immediately to the emergency room. What is a possible explanation for why her child is experiencing these symptoms? What is the causative agent for these symptoms? Is this a serious threat to her child?

30. Dr. Harry is a pediatrician who recently examined a 2-year-old boy who awakened in the middle of the night frightened and with the following symptoms: labored inspiration, harsh and vibrating cough, and a normal body temperature. What diagnosis might Dr. Harry give his patient? Is this life-threatening?

31. Mr. Gorski is a heavy smoker. Recently, he has noticed that when he gets up in the morning, he has a bothersome cough that brings up a large accumulation of mucus. This cough persists for several minutes and then leaves until the next morning. What is a possible explanation for this problem?

DID YOU KNOW ?

- If the roof of your mouth is narrow, you are more likely to snore since you are not getting enough oxygen through your nose.

- Only about 10% of the air in the lungs is actually changed with each cycle of inhaling and exhaling when an at-rest person is breathing, but up to 80% can be exchanged during deep breathing or strenuous exercise.

ONE LAST QUICK CHECK ✓

Matching—choose the correct response.

a. nose
b. pharynx
c. larynx

32. _____ warms and humidifies air

33. _____ air and food pass through here

34. _____ sinuses

35. _____ conchae

36. _____ septum

37. _____ tonsils

38. _____ middle ear infections

39. _____ epiglottis

40. _____ rhinitis

41. _____ sore throat

42. _____ epistaxis

Fill in the blanks.

The organs of the respiratory system are designed to perform two basic functions. They serve as an
(43) _____
_____ and as a
(44) _____ _____. In addition to the above, the respiratory system
(45) _____,
(46) _____, and
(47) _____ the air we breathe. Respiratory organs include the
(48) _____,
(49) _____,
(50) _____,
(51) _____,
(52) _____, and the
(53) _____. The respiratory system ends in millions of tiny, thin-walled sacs called
(54) _____.
(55) _____ of gases takes place in these sacs. Two aspects of the structure of these sacs assist them in the exchange of gases. First, an extremely thin membrane, the
(56) _____ _____, allows for easy exchange and second, the large number of air sacs makes an enormous
(57) _____ area.

CHAPTER 24

Physiology of the Respiratory System

The respiratory system functions to diffuse gases into and out of the blood so that the organs of our body receive blood that is rich in oxygen and low in carbon dioxide. The exchange of gases that occurs within the body is a complex operation and each component of the pulmonary system contributes to successful ventilation. Air must enter the lungs (inspiration) from the external environment, an exchange must occur between the blood and the cells, and then air high in CO_2 is returned to the environment (expiration).

Numerous anatomical and physiological mechanisms influence the successful exchange of gases throughout the process. The rate, depth, and pressure of pulmonary ventilation are dependent upon these structures to successfully perform their respiratory function. Your review of this system is necessary to provide you with an understanding of this essential homeostatic mechanism necessary for survival.

I—PULMONARY VENTILATION

Multiple Choice—select the best answer.

1. Boyle's law states that:
   a. fluids move from areas of high pressure to low.
   b. the volume of a gas is inversely proportional to its pressure.
   c. the atmosphere exerts a pressure of 760 mm Hg.
   d. volume is directly proportional to temperature.

2. When the diaphragm contracts, the volume of the thorax increases, thoracic pressure:
   a. increases, and air is forced from the lungs.
   b. decreases, and air is forced from the lungs.
   c. decreases, and air rushes into the lungs.
   d. increases, and air rushes into the lungs.

3. Quiet inspiration is the function of:
   a. the diaphragm and internal intercostal.
   b. the diaphragm and external intercostal.
   c. the internal intercostal and external intercostal.
   d. none of the above.

4. During normal, quiet respiration, the amount of air exchanged between the lungs and atmosphere is called _____ and has a volume of _____ ml.
   a. tidal volume; 1200 ml
   b. vital capacity; 4500 ml
   c. tidal volume; 500 ml
   d. residual volume; 1200 ml

5. Functional residual capacity (FRC) equals:
   a. TV + IRV.
   b. TV + IRV + ERV + RV.
   c. TV + IRV + ERV.
   d. ERV + RV.

6. *Eupnea* is a term used to describe:
   a. rapid, deep respiration.
   b. cessation of respiration.
   c. slow, shallow respiration.
   d. normal breathing.

7. Under normal conditions, air in the atmosphere exerts a pressure of:
   a. 500 mm Hg.
   b. 560 mm Hg.
   c. 660 mm Hg.
   d. 760 mm Hg.

8. Areas where gas exchange cannot take place are:
   a. anatomical dead spaces.
   b. nose, pharynx, larynx.
   c. trachea and bronchi.
   d. all of the above.

9. All of the following are regulated processes associated with the functioning of the respiratory system *EXCEPT*:
   a. control of cell reproduction.
   b. gas exchange in lungs and tissue.
   c. pulmonary ventilation.
   d. transport of gases.

10. Dalton's law is also known as:
    a. Henry's law.
    b. Boyle's law.
    c. Charles' law.
    d. the law of partial pressures.

True or false

11. _____ Temperature is the measurement of the motion of molecules.

12. _____ The largest amount of air that can enter and leave the lungs during respiration is termed *total lung capacity (TLC)*.

13. _____ Residual volume (RV) is the volume remaining in the respiratory tract after maximum expiration.

14. _____ The temporary cessation of breathing is termed *apnea*.

15. _____ It is not possible to exhale all of the air from your lungs.

Labeling—label the following diagram with the correct terminology for the lung volumes displayed.

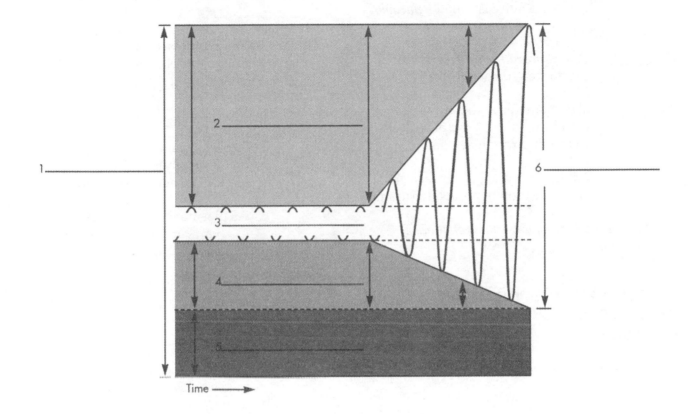

Time ⟶

▷ *If you had difficulty with this section, review pages 884-899.*

II—PULMONARY GAS EXCHANGE

Multiple Choice—select the best answer.

16. If oxygen is 21% of the atmosphere, it will contribute _____ of the total atmospheric pressure.
    a. 21%
    b. 79%
    c. 0.21%
    d. .79%

17. The amount of oxygen that diffuses into blood each minute depends on the:
    a. total functional surface area of the respiratory membrane.
    b. respiratory minute volume.
    c. alveolar ventilation.
    d. all of the above.

18. P_{O_2} at standard atmospheric pressure is approximately:
    a. 21 mm Hg.
    b. 0.2 mm Hg.
    c. 160 mm Hg.
    d. 760 mm Hg.

19. Anything that decreases the total functional surface area of the respiratory membrane:
    a. tends to decrease oxygen diffusion into the blood.
    b. tends to increase oxygen diffusion into the blood.
    c. has little effect on oxygen diffusion.
    d. increases the humidity of oxygen as it diffuses.

True or false

20. _____ Air in the pleural space of the thoracic cavity is called a *pneumothorax.*

21. _____ *Partial pressure* and *tension* can be used interchangeably.

22. _____ The diameter of the pulmonary capillaries allows red blood cells to travel through at 10 abreast.

23. _____ Nitrogen is the gas of greatest concentration in atmospheric air.

▷ *If you had difficulty with this section, review pages 899-903.*

III—BLOOD TRANSPORTATION OF GASES AND SYSTEMIC GAS EXCHANGE

Multiple Choice—select the best answer.

24. Oxygen is carried in blood:
    a. as oxyhemoglobin.
    b. dissolved in plasma.
    c. molecularly as HbO_2.
    d. all of the above.

25. Which of the following is *NOT* a manner in which CO_2 is transported in the blood?
    a. dissolved in plasma
    b. bound to the heme group of the hemoglobin molecule
    c. as bicarbonate ions
    d. bound to the polypeptide chains of hemoglobin

26. Increasing the carbon dioxide content of blood results in:
    a. increased H^+ concentration of plasma.
    b. decreased blood pH.
    c. increased blood pH.
    d. both a and b.
    e. both a and c.

27. Approximately 97% of oxygen is transported as _____, whereas the remaining 3% is transported dissolved in _____.
    a. plasma; hemoglobin
    b. oxyhemoglobin; bicarbonate ion
    c. oxyhemoglobin; plasma
    d. bicarbonate ion; carbonic acid

True or false

28. _____ The exact amount of oxygen in blood depends mainly upon the amount of hemoglobin present.

29. _____ As plasma P_{CO_2} increases, the CO_2 carrying capacity of blood decreases.

30. _____ Interstitial fluid P_{O_2} and intracellular fluid P_{O_2} are essentially the same.

31. _____ A right shift of the oxygen-hemoglobin dissociation curve due to increased P_{CO_2} is known as the *Bohr effect.*

▷ *If you had difficulty with this section, review pages 903-910.*

IV—REGULATION OF BREATHING

Multiple Choice—select the best answer.

32. The basic rhythm of the respiratory cycle seems to be generated by:
    a. the medullary rhythmicity area.
    b. the inspiratory center.
    c. the expiratory center.
    d. all of the above.

33. The diving reflex:
    a. explains why some people can hold their breath for extended periods while under water.
    b. is responsible for the astonishing recovery of near-drowning victims in cold water.
    c. forces a submerged individual to exhale prior to surfacing.
    d. both a and c.

True or false

34. _____ Input from the apneustic center in the pons inhibits the inspiratory center, causing a decrease in the length and depth of inspiration.

35. _____ Irritation of the phrenic nerve can cause extended periods of hiccups.

Labeling—using the terms provided, label the respiratory centers of the brainstem on the following illustration.

medulla
expiratory area
apneustic center
inspiratory center
respiratory centers

pons
pneumotaxic center
cortex
limbic system
respiratory muscles

1 _____
2 _____
3 _____
4 _____
5 _____
6 _____
7 _____
8 _____

9 _____

10 _____

▷ *If you had difficulty with this section, review pages 912-916.*

V—MECHANISMS OF DISEASE

Fill in the blanks.

36. _____ or _____ _____ _____ is a broad term used to describe conditions of progressive, irreversible obstruction of expiratory air flow.

37. _____ results from excessive tracheobronchial secretions that obstruct air flow.

38. _____ may result from the progression of chronic bronchitis or other conditions as air becomes trapped within alveoli causing them to enlarge and eventually rupture.

39. _____ is an obstructive disorder characterized by recurring spasms of the smooth muscle in the walls of the bronchial air passages.

▷ *If you had difficulty with this section, review pages 916-919.*

Crossword Puzzle

Across
2. Labored breathing
6. Inhaling
7. Volume of air exhaled after inspiration (two words)
8. Most carbon dioxide is carried in this form
9. Hemoglobin combined with oxygen

Down
1. "Tension" (two words)
3. Used to measure amount of air exchanged in breathing
4. Exhaling
5. Breathing

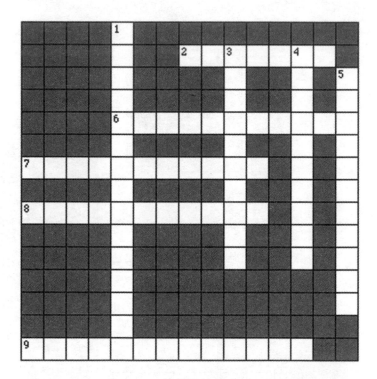

APPLYING WHAT YOU KNOW

40. Mr. Gaines has smoked a considerable number of cigars and cigarettes during the last two decades. He is beginning to have difficulty breathing—especially upon exhalation. Which broad category of diseases may he be exhibiting symptoms of? What other diseases is he at risk for? What are the physiological mechanisms of these diseases?

41. While sledding on a frozen creek, Heather, a 12-year-old girl, fell through the ice. Her situation wasn't discovered for about half an hour. Upon rescue, she displayed fixed, dilated pupils; cyanosis; and no pulse. Miraculously, she recovered. Identify and explain the physiological phenomena that resulted in this astonishing recovery.

DID YOU KNOW ?

- Sinusitis affects 37 million Americans causing difficulty in breathing and chronic headaches.

- A person's nose and ears continue to grow throughout his or her life.

ONE LAST QUICK CHECK ✔

Multiple Choice—select the best answer.

42. The term that means the same thing as *breathing* is:
    a. gas exchange.
    b. respiration.
    c. inspiration.
    d. pulmonary ventilation.

43. Carbaminohemoglobin is formed when _____ bind(s) to hemoglobin.
    a. oxygen
    b. amino acids
    c. carbon dioxide
    d. nitrogen

44. Most of the oxygen transported by the blood is:
    a. dissolved to white blood cells.
    b. bound to white blood cells.
    c. bound to hemoglobin.
    d. bound to carbaminohemoglobin.

45. Which of the following does *NOT* occur during inspiration?
    a. elevation of the ribs
    b. the diaphragm relaxes
    c. alveolar pressure decreases
    d. chest cavity becomes longer from top to bottom

46. A young adult male would have a vital capacity of about _____ ml.
    a. 500
    b. 1200
    c. 3300
    d. 4800

47. The amount of air that can be forcibly exhaled after expiring the tidal volume is known as the:
    a. total lung capacity.
    b. vital capacity.
    c. inspiratory reserve volume.
    d. expiratory reserve volume.

48. Which one of the following is correct?
    a. VC = TV – IRV + ERV
    b. VC = TV + IRV – ERV
    c. VC = TV + IRV x ERV
    d. VC = TV + IRV + ERV

Matching—identify the term with the proper selection.

a. collapsed lung
b. quaternary protein
c. approximately 3300 ml
d. Po_2
e. normal exhalation volume
f. increased in emphysema
g. helps control respirations
h. respiratory stimulant
i. cessation of breathing
j. sensitive to changes in arterial CO_2 and pH

49. _____ tidal volume

50. _____ inspiratory reserve volume

51. _____ pneumothorax

52. _____ physiological dead space

53. _____ oxygen tension

54. _____ hemoglobin

55. _____ apneusis

56. _____ chemoreceptors

57. _____ Hering-Breuer reflexes

58. _____ CO_2

CHAPTER 25

Anatomy of the Digestive System

Think of the last meal you ate. The different shapes, sizes, tastes, and textures that you so recently enjoyed. Think of those items circulating in your bloodstream in those same original shapes and sizes. Impossible? Of course. Because of this impossibility you can begin to understand and marvel at the close relationship of the digestive system to the circulatory system. It is the digestive system that changes our food, both mechanically and chemically, into a form that is acceptable to the blood and the body.

This change begins the moment you take the very first bite. Digestion starts in the mouth, where food is chewed and mixed with saliva. It then moves down the pharynx and esophagus by peristalsis and enters the stomach. In the stomach it is churned and mixed with gastric juices to continue the digestive process. As the food continues into the small intestine, it is further broken down chemically by intestinal fluids, bile, and pancreatic juice. These secretions prepare the food for absorption all along the course of the small intestine (duodenum, jejunum, and ileum). Products that are not absorbed pass on and enter the cecum of the large intestine and continue through the ascending colon, transverse colon, descending colon, sigmoid colon, into the rectum, and out the anus.

Products that are used in the cells undergo absorption. Absorption allows newly processed nutrients to pass through the walls of the digestive tract and into the bloodstream to be distributed to the cells. Your review of this system will help you understand the anatomy that provides the mechanical and chemical processes necessary to convert food into energy sources and compounds necessary for survival.

I—OVERVIEW OF THE DIGESTIVE SYSTEM

Multiple Choice—select the best answer.

1. Starting from the deepest layer and moving towards the most superficial, the layers of the wall of the GI tract are:
   a. mucosa, submucosa, serosa, muscularis.
   b. submucosa, mucosa, muscularis, serosa.
   c. mucosa, submucosa, muscularis, serosa.
   d. submucosa, serosa, muscularis, mucosa.

2. The serosa is actually:
    a. parietal peritoneum.
    b. visceral peritoneum.
    c. mesentery.
    d. none of the above.

True or false

3. _____   *Gastrointestinal tract* and *alimentary canal* are synonymous terms.

4. _____   The tissue layers of the GI tract are constant, with no variation in the different organs.

Matching—identify each digestive organ with its correct classification.

a. GI tract segment   b. accessory organ

5. _____   mouth

6. _____   jejunum

7. _____   cecum

8. _____   pancreas

9. _____   teeth

10. _____   liver

11. _____   salivary glands

12. _____   vermiform appendix

13. _____   oropharynx

14. _____   sigmoid colon

Labeling—label the digestive organs on the following illustration.

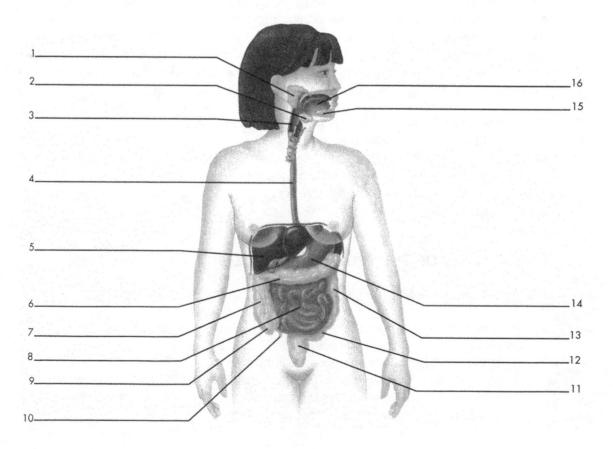

If you had difficulty with this section, review pages 926-928.

II—MOUTH AND PHARYNX

Multiple Choice—select the best answer.

15. The hard palate consists of portions of:
    a. three bones: two maxillae and one palatine.
    b. two bones: one maxillae and one palatine.
    c. three bones: one maxillae and two palatine.
    d. four bones: two maxillae and two palatine.

16. Which of the following is an accurate description of salivary glands?
    a. There are four pairs of salivary glands.
    b. They secrete about one liter of saliva per day.
    c. They are associated with buccal glands that secrete about 50% of the saliva.
    d. Both b and c are true.

17. The crown of a tooth is covered with:
    a. dentin.
    b. cementum.
    c. enamel.
    d. alveolar bone.

18. The type of teeth that do *NOT* appear as deciduous teeth are:
    a. incisors.
    b. canines.
    c. second molars.
    d. premolars.

19. The act of swallowing moves a mass of food called a _____ from the mouth to the stomach.
    a. dentin
    b. bolus
    c. fauces
    d. philtrum

True or false

20. __T__   A typical tooth can be divided into three main parts: crown, neck, and root.

21. _____   The *philtrum* is a fold of mucous membrane that helps anchor the tongue to the floor of the mouth.

22. _____   There are 20 deciduous teeth and 30 permanent teeth.

23. _____   The act of swallowing is termed *deglutition*.

24. _____   The soft palate forms a partition between the mouth and oropharynx.

Labeling—label the structures of the tooth on the following illustration.

▷ *If you had difficulty with this section, review pages 929-934.*

III—ESOPHAGUS AND STOMACH

Multiple Choice—select the best answer.

25. Which of the following statements is *NOT* true of the esophagus?
    a. It extends from the pharynx to the stomach.
    b. It lies anterior to the trachea and posterior to the heart.
    c. It resides in both the thoracic and abdominal cavities.
    d. It pierces the diaphragm.

26. Which of the following controls the opening of the stomach into the small intestine?
    a. pylorus
    b. cardiac sphincter
    c. duodenal bulb
    d. pyloric sphincter

27. Which of the layers of the muscularis is present only in the stomach?
    a. longitudinal muscle layer
    b. circular muscle layer
    c. oblique muscle layer
    d. horizontal muscle layer

True or false

28. _____ The folds in the lining of the stomach are called *rugae*.

29. _____ The cardiac sphincter controls the opening of the esophagus into the stomach.

30. _____ Parietal cells secrete hydrochloric acid and are thought to produce intrinsic factor.

Labeling—using the terms provided, label the following illustration of the stomach.

fundus   pylorus   pyloric sphincter
duodenal bulb   cardiac sphincter   oblique muscle layer
serosa   submucosa   body
esophagus   longitudinal muscle layer   circular muscle layer
lesser curvature   greater curvature   gastroesophageal opening
duodenum   mucosa   rugae

1. _____
2. _____
3. _____
4. _____
5. _____
6. _____
7. _____
8. _____
9. _____

18 _____
17 _____
16 _____
15 _____
14 _____
13 _____
12 _____
11 _____
10 _____

 If you had difficulty with this section, review pages 934-938.

IV—SMALL INTESTINE, LARGE INTESTINE, APPENDIX, AND PERITONEUM

Multiple Choice—select the best answer.

31. The correct order of small intestine divisions, starting proximal to the stomach, is:
    a. ileum, duodenum, jejunum.
    b. duodenum, ileum, jejunum.
    c. duodenum, jejunum, ileum.
    d. ileum, jejunum, duodenum.

32. Beginning with the largest structures, which of the following is a correct description of the small intestine's adaptation for absorption?
    a. villi, microvilli, plicae
    b. plicae, villi, microvilli
    c. microvilli, villi, plicae
    d. microvilli, plicae, villi

33. Another term for hemorrhoids is:
    a. piles.
    b. fistula.
    c. fissures.
    d. proctitis.

34. The lesser omentum attaches the:
    a. transverse colon to the posterior abdominal wall.
    b. liver to the lesser curvature of the stomach.
    c. ileum and jejunum to the posterior abdominal wall.
    d. greater omentum to the posterior abdominal wall.

True or false

35. _____ The hepatic flexure of the large intestine is also called the *left colic flexure.*

36. _____ The nonpathogenic bacteria of the colon are thought to be produced in the sigmoid colon.

37. __T___ The pouchlike structures of the large intestine are called *haustra.*

38. __T___ Hemorrhoids are enlargements of veins in the anal canal.

Labeling—label the wall of the small intestine on the following illustration.

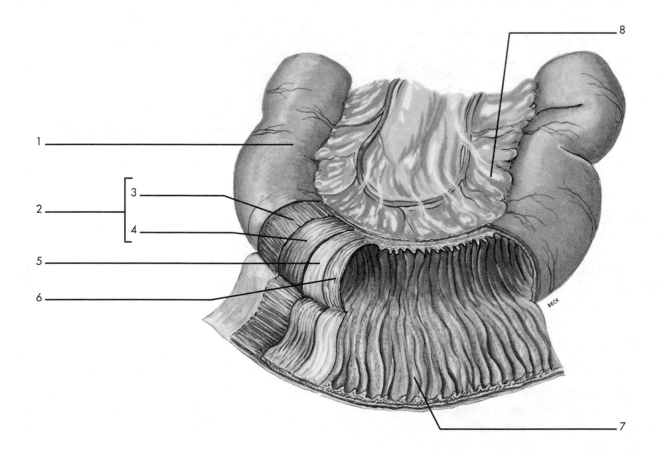

Labeling—label the divisions of the large intestine on the following illustration.

▷ *If you had difficulty with this section, review pages 939-944.*

V—LIVER, GALLBLADDER, AND PANCREAS

Multiple Choice—select the best answer.

39. The anatomical units of the liver are called:
    a. lobes.
    b. lobules.
    c. sinusoids.
    d. none of the above.

40. Blood flows to hepatic lobules via branches of the:
    a. hepatic artery.
    b. hepatic portal vein.
    c. hepatic vein.
    d. both a and b.

41. A merger of the hepatic duct and cystic duct form the:
    a. common hepatic duct.
    b. common bile duct.
    c. right hepatic duct.
    d. left hepatic duct.

42. Bile salts aid in the absorption of:
    a. fat.
    b. carbohydrates.
    c. proteins.
    d. waste products.

True or false

43. ___T___ The liver consists of two lobes separated by the falciform ligament.

44. ___F___ Bile is manufactured by the Kupffer cells of the liver.

45. ___T___ The pancreas is both an endocrine and exocrine gland.

46. ___T___ Surgical removal of the gallbladder is called *cholecystectomy*.

Labeling—label the gross structure of the liver on the following illustration.

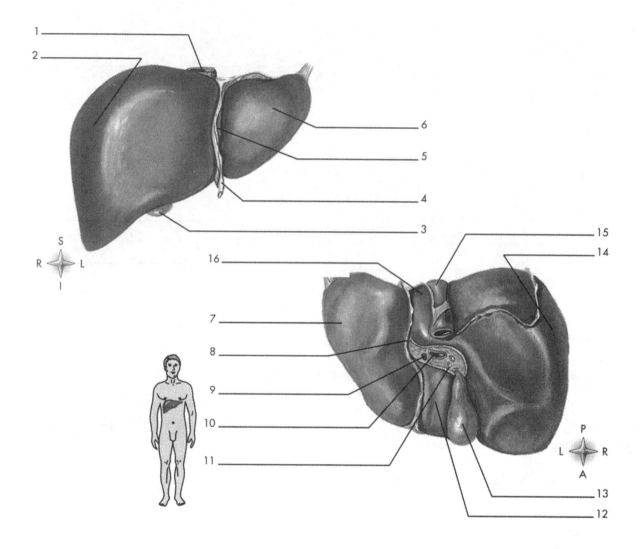

Labeling—label the ducts on the following illustration of the common bile duct and its tributaries.

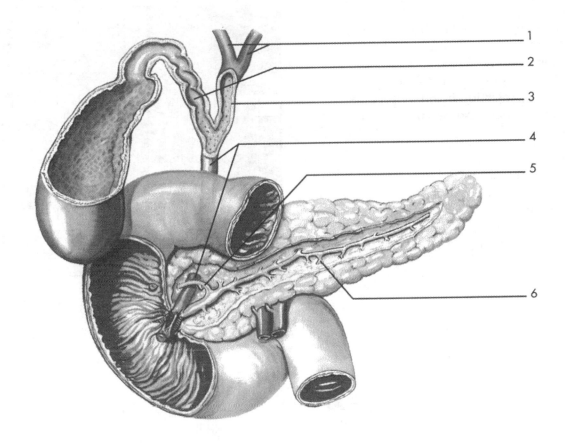

1
2
3
4
5
6

▷ *If you had difficulty with this section, review pages 944-950.*

VI—MECHANISMS OF DISEASE

Matching—identify the term with the appropriate description.

a. corrects malocclusion
b. swelling of parotid glands
c. inflammation of rectal mucosa
d. dilated veins
e. autoimmune disease that targets salivary and tear glands
f. obstructive narrowing
g. low incidence in elderly
h. minor laceration
i. causes most gastric and duodenal ulcers
j. gastric reflux
k. infection of gums

47. _____ hemorrhoids
48. _____ appendicitis
49. _____ pyloric stenosis
50. _____ Sjögren's syndrome
51. _____ *Helicobacter pylori*
52. _____ orthodontics
53. _____ anal fissures
54. _____ mumps
55. _____ proctitis
56. _____ gingivitis
57. _____ heartburn

▷ *If you had difficulty with this section, review pages 951-955.*

Crossword Puzzle

Across

1. Alimentary canal (abbrev., two words)
3. Stored in gallbladder
5. Division of small intestine
8. Small projection in small intestine
9. Large sheet of serous membrane
11. Chewing

Down

2. Large intestine
4. First segment of digestive tube
6. Swallowing
7. Refers to liver
10. Innermost layer of GI tract

APPLYING WHAT YOU KNOW

58. Brian is experiencing difficulty digesting fatty foods and is displaying a yellow discoloration of his skin. What may be causing his condition? What is the clinical term used to describe the yellow appearance of his skin and what is the physiology? How could doctors treat his condition and what are the names of the procedures?

59. Baby Billy has been regurgitating his bottle feeding at every meal. The milk is curdled, but does not appear to be digested. He has become dehydrated, so his mother, Amanda, is taking him to the pediatrician. What is a possible diagnosis from your textbook reading?

DID YOU KNOW

- The human stomach lining replaces itself every 3 days.

- If one were to unravel the entire human alimentary canal (esophagus, stomach, small and large intestines), it would reach the height of a three-story building.

ONE LAST QUICK CHECK

Multiple Choice—select the best answer.

60. The first baby tooth, on an average, appears at age:
    a. 2 months.
    b. 1 year.
    c. 1 month.
    d. 6 months.

61. The portion of the tooth that is covered with enamel is the:
    a. pulp cavity.
    b. neck.
    c. root.
    d. crown.

62. Which of the following teeth is missing from the deciduous arch?
    a. central incisor
    b. canine
    c. second premolar
    d. first molar

63. The permanent central incisor erupts between the ages of _____.
    a. 9 and 13
    b. 5 and 6
    c. 7 and 10
    d. 7 and 8

64. A general term for infection of the gums is:
    a. dental caries.
    b. leukoplakia.
    c. Vincent's angina.
    d. gingivitis.

65. The ducts of the _____ glands open into the floor of the mouth.
    a. sublingual
    b. submandibular
    c. parotid
    d. carotid

66. The volume of saliva secreted per day is about:
    a. 1/2 pint.
    b. 1 pint.
    c. 1 liter.
    d. 1 gallon.

67. Another name for the third molar is:
    a. central incisor.
    b. wisdom tooth.
    c. canine.
    d. lateral incisor.

68. After food has been chewed, it is formed into a small rounded mass called a:
    a. moat.
    b. chyme.
    c. bolus.
    d. protease.

69. Which one is *NOT* part of the small intestine?
    a. jejunum
    b. ileum
    c. cecum
    d. duodenum

70. The union of the cystic duct and hepatic duct forms the:
    a. common bile duct.
    b. major duodenal papilla.
    c. minor duodenal papilla.
    d. pancreatic duct.

71. Each villus in the intestine contains a lymphatic vessel or _____ that serves to absorb lipid or fat materials from the chyme.
    a. plica
    b. lacteal
    c. villa
    d. microvilli

72. *Cholelithiasis* is the term used to describe:
    a. biliary colic.
    b. jaundice.
    c. portal hypertension.
    d. gallstones.

73. The largest gland in the body is the:
    a. pituitary.
    b. thyroid.
    c. liver.
    d. thymus.

True or false

74. _____ The splenic flexure is the bend between the ascending colon and the transverse colon.

75. _____ The splenic colon is the S-shaped segment that terminates in the rectum.

76. _____ The function of the appendix is uncertain.

77. _____ The oral cavity is also known as the *buccal cavity.*

78. _____ The esophagus is voluntary in the upper third, mixed in the middle, and involuntary in the lower third.

79. _____ The stomach secretes the intrinsic factor.

80. _____ The mesentery is a fan-shaped projection of the parietal peritoneum.

81. _____ The first step in the digestive process is called *mechanical digestion* and the second phase of digestion is called *chemical digestion.*

82. _____ The fundus, pylorus, and plicae are the three main divisions of the stomach.

CHAPTER 26

Physiology of the Digestive System

D igestion is the process of breaking down complex nutrients into simpler units suitable for absorption. It involves two major processes: mechanical and chemical. Mechanical digestion occurs during mastication and the churning and propelling mechanisms that take place along the alimentary canal. Chemical digestion occurs with the help of the many digestive enzymes and various substances that are added to the nutrients as they progress the length of the digestive tube. These substances include saliva and gastric, pancreatic, and intestinal enzymes. Delicate nervous and hormonal reflex mechanisms control the flow of these juices so that the proper amount is released at the appropriate time.

Absorption is the passage of substances (digested foods, water, salts, and vitamins) through the intestinal mucosa and into the blood or lymph. After the body has determined the nutrients necessary for absorption, it sends the residue of digestion to the final segment of the GI tract to be eliminated as feces.

Your review of this system will help you understand the mechanical and chemical processes necessary to convert food into energy sources and compounds necessary for survival.

I—DIGESTION

Multiple Choice—select the best answer.

1. Which of the following describes the pharyngeal stage of deglutition?
   a. mouth to oropharynx
   b. oropharynx to esophagus
   c. esophagus to stomach
   d. none of the above

2. Which step of deglutition is under voluntary control?
   a. oral
   b. pharyngeal
   c. esophageal
   d. all of the above

3. The final product of carbohydrate digestion is a:
   a. disaccharide.
   b. monosaccharide.
   c. polysaccharide.
   d. fatty acid.

4. Enzymes that catalyze the hydrolysis of proteins are:
   a. proteases.
   b. amylases.
   c. lactases.
   d. lipases.

5. A micelle is:
   a. a disaccharide attached to the brush border of the small intestine.
   b. a tiny sphere of lipid and water.
   c. a thick, milky material comprised of food and digestive enzymes.
   d. synonymous with *bolus*.

6. Which of the following is *NOT* true concerning the gastric emptying of water?
   a. Large volumes of water leave the stomach more rapidly than small volumes.
   b. Warm fluids empty more quickly than cool fluids.
   c. High-solute concentration fluids empty slower than dilute concentrations.
   d. All of the above are true.

7. The process of fat emulsification consists of:
   a. chemically breaking down fat molecules.
   b. absorption of fats.
   c. breaking down fats into small droplets.
   d. the secretion of digestive juices for fat digestion.

True or false

8. ___F___   Peristalsis can be described as a mixing movement.

9. ___F___   The volumes of the stomach and the duodenum are approximately equal.

   ___T___

10. _____   Enzymes are organic catalysts.

11. _____   Digestive enzymes catalyze chemical reactions with great efficiency within a wide range of pH.

12. ___F___   Cellulose resists digestion and is eliminated in feces.

13. ___F___   Water is readily absorbed in the stomach.

14. ___T___   Amino acids are the end product of protein digestion.

▶ *If you had difficulty with this section, review pages 962-973.*

II—SECRETION AND CONTROL OF DIGESTIVE GLAND SECRETION

Multiple Choice—select the best answer.

15. The principal enzyme of saliva is:
    a. protease.
    b. amylase.
    c. lipase.
    d. salivase.

16. Which of the following is true?
    a. Saliva contains large amounts of lipase.
    b. Pepsinogen is converted into pepsin by hydrochloric acid.
    c. Chief cells secrete pepsin.
    d. Zymogenic cells produce intrinsic factor.

17. Which of the following is present in bile?
    a. lecithin
    b. gastrin
    c. bile salts
    d. both a and c

18. The hormone that stimulates the gallbladder to release bile is:
    a. enterogastrone.
    b. insulin.
    c. gastrin.
    d. cholecystokinin.

True or false

19. ___T___ Pancreatic juice is secreted by exocrine acinar cells of the pancreas.

20. ___T___ Olfactory and visual stimuli are factors concerning the control of digestive gland secretion.

21. ___F___ The cephalic phase is initiated by the presence of food in the stomach.

22. ___T___ Chyme is liquefied food found in the stomach.

▶ *If you had difficulty with this section, review pages 973-980.*

III—ABSORPTION AND ELIMINATION

Multiple Choice—select the best answer.

23. Fats are absorbed primarily into which of the following structures?
    a. blood in intestinal capillaries
    b. lymph in intestinal lacteals
    c. none of the above

24. Movement of lower colon and rectum contents at a rate slower than normal can cause:
    a. defecation.
    b. constipation.
    c. diarrhea.
    d. both b and c.

25. Which blood vessel carries absorbed nutrients from the GI tract to the liver?
    a. hepatic artery
    b. hepatic vein
    c. portal vein
    d. inferior vena cava

True or false

26. _____ Both water and sodium are absorbed via simple diffusion.

27. _____ The majority of substances are absorbed in the small intestine.

28. _____ Cholera is an intestinal infection that kills more than 600,000 infants and children worldwide each year.

29. _____ Micelles, formed from bile salts, carry fatty acids from emulsified droplets to the plasma membrane of absorptive cells.

30. _____ Impaired fat absorption produces large, greasy, foul-smelling stools known as *steatorrhea*.

▶ *If you had difficulty with this section, review pages 980-984.*

IV—MECHANISMS OF DISEASE

Matching—select the best term for the description.

a. reduces the formation of HCl in the stomach
b. outpouchings of the intestinal wall
c. inflammation of the liver
d. chronic loss of appetite
e. degenerative liver condition
f. cause of ulcers
g. vomiting
h. stomach inflammation
i. inflammation of large intestine
j. a form of adenocarcinoma

31. _____ gastroenteritis

32. _____ anorexia

33. _____ emesis

34. _____ Zantac

35. _____ *Helicobacter pylori*

36. _____ diverticulosis

37. _____ colitis

38. _____ hepatitis

39. _____ pancreatic cancer

40. _____ cirrhosis

▶ *If you had difficulty with this section, review pages 985-988.*

Crossword Puzzle

Across

5. Process of taking food into the GI tract
6. Food leaving the stomach
7. Mixing movement
9. GI hormones
10. Chemical process in digestion

Down

1. Wavelike ripple of organ
2. Fat droplet
3. Expelling feces
4. Fat droplet surrounded by bile salts
8. Movement of nutrients into internal environment

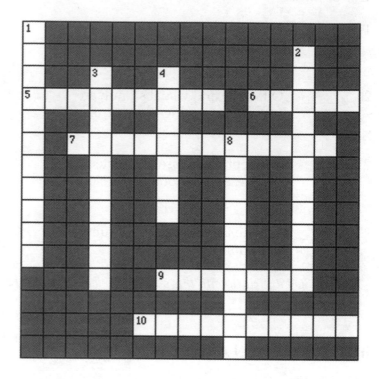

APPLYING WHAT YOU KNOW

41. Mrs. Haygood was diagnosed with an ulcer of the digestive system. What kind of symptoms might she display? Where along her alimentary canal is this lesion most likely to reside? What are the two accepted mechanisms of this disease? How should her doctor treat her condition?

42. Cliff and Pete like to play soccer vigorously in the heat of the day. What kind of recommendations should they observe concerning the replacement of fluids? Be sure to consider parameters such as fluid temperature, volume, and solute concentration.

DID YOU KNOW ?

- There are 35 million digestive glands in the stomach.

- Even if the stomach, the spleen, 75% of the liver, 80% of the intestines, one kidney, one lung, and virtually every organ from the pelvic and groin area are removed, the human body can still survive!

ONE LAST QUICK CHECK ✔

Multiple Choice—select the best answer.

43. During the process of digestion, stored bile is poured into the duodenum by which of the following?
    a. gallbladder
    b. liver
    c. pancreas
    d. spleen

44. The portion of the alimentary canal that mixes food with gastric juice and breaks it down into a mixture called *chyme* is the:
    a. gallbladder.
    b. small intestine.
    c. stomach.
    d. large intestine.

45. What is the middle portion of the small intestine called?
    a. jejunum
    b. ileum
    c. duodenum
    d. cecum

46. Duodenal ulcers appear in which of the following?
    a. stomach
    b. small intestine
    c. large intestine
    d. esophagus

47. Protein digestion begins in the:
    a. esophagus.
    b. small intestine.
    c. stomach.
    d. large intestine.

48. The enzyme pepsin is concerned primarily with the digestion of which of the following?
    a. sugars
    b. starches
    c. proteins
    d. fats

49. The enzyme amylase converts which of the following?
    a. starches to sugars
    b. sugars to starches
    c. proteins to amino acids
    d. fatty acids and glycerols to fats

50. Which of the following substances does NOT contain any enzymes?
    a. saliva
    b. bile
    c. gastric juice
    d. intestinal juice

51. Which of the following is a simple sugar?
    a. maltose
    b. sucrose
    c. lactose
    d. glucose

52. Fats are broken down into:
    a. amino acids.
    b. simple sugars.
    c. fatty acids.
    d. disaccharides.

53. Which one is NOT part of the small intestine?
    a. jejunum
    b. ileum
    c. colon
    d. duodenum

54. The union of the cystic duct and hepatic duct form the:
    a. common bile duct.
    b. major duodenal papilla.
    c. minor duodenal papilla.
    d. pancreatic duct.

55. The process of swallowing is known as:
    a. mastication.
    b. segmentation.
    c. peristalsis.
    d. deglutition.

56. Peristalsis begins in the:
    a. mouth.
    b. pharynx.
    c. esophagus.
    d. stomach.

True or false

57. _____ The mechanical process that occurs in the rectum is churning.

58. _____ Enzymes are functional proteins that catalyze chemical reactions.

59. _____ The hormones secretin and CCK stimulate ejection of bile.

60. _____ Vitamins A, D, E, and K are known as the *fat-soluble vitamins*.

61. _____ Constipation occurs with increased motility of the small intestine.

CHAPTER 27

Nutrition and Metabolism

Most of us love to eat, but do the foods we enjoy provide us with the basic food types necessary for good nutrition? The body, a finely tuned machine, requires a balance of carbohydrates, fats, proteins, vitamins, and minerals to function properly. These nutrients must be digested, absorbed, and circulated to cells constantly to accommodate the numerous activities that occur throughout the body. The use the body makes of foods once these processes are completed is called "metabolism."

Although the body relies on many organs to prepare nutrients, the liver plays a major role in the metabolism of food. It helps maintain a normal blood glucose level, removes toxins from the blood, processes blood immediately after it leaves the gastrointestinal tract, and initiates the first steps of protein and fat metabolism.

The study of metabolism is not complete without a discussion of the basal metabolic rate (BMR). The BMR is the rate at which food is catabolized under basal conditions. The total metabolic rate (TMR) is the amount of energy, expressed in calories, used by the body each day. This chapter also demonstrates the use of metabolic testing to measure thyroid functioning.

Finally, the hypothalamus appears to be a critical component in determining appetite and satiety. While many theories suggest various ways that the hypothalamus might perform these functions, it is imperative that we acknowledge its importance in nutrition and metabolism. Review of this chapter is necessary to provide you with an understanding of the "fuel," or nutrition, necessary to maintain your complex homeostatic machine—the body.

I—OVERVIEW OF NUTRITION AND METABOLISM

Multiple Choice—select the best answer.

1. The universal biological currency is:
   a. ATP.
   b. ADP.
   c. carbohydrates.
   d. NADH.

2. *Nutrition* refers to the:
   a. complex set of chemical processes that make life possible.
   b. breaking down of food into small molecular compounds.
   c. release of energy in two main forms.
   d. food we eat and the nutrients they contain.

True or false

3. _____ Catabolism is a process that breaks down molecules into smaller molecular compounds.

4. _____ Metabolism is identical in all cells.

▷ *If you had difficulty with this section, review pages 994-996.*

II—CARBOHYDRATES

Multiple Choice—select the best answer.

5. Glucose, fructose, and galactose are important:
   a. monosaccharides.
   b. disaccharides.
   c. polysaccharides.
   d. starches.

6. The carbohydrate most useful to the human cell is:
   a. cellulose.
   b. glucose.
   c. fructose.
   d. galactose.

7. The process of glucose phosphorylation forms the molecule:
   a. ATP.
   b. ADP.
   c. glucose-6-phosphate.
   d. glycogen.

8. The breakdown of one glucose molecule into two pyruvic acid molecules is called:
   a. glycolysis.
   b. glycogenesis.
   c. glycogenolysis.
   d. glycogen.

9. The amount of heat necessary to raise the temperature of 1 g of water by 1° C is a:
   a. calorie.
   b. Celsius.
   c. kilocalorie.
   d. none of the above.

10. To enter the citric acid cycle, glucose must be transformed into:
    a. pyruvic acid.
    b. acetyl-CoA.
    c. ATP.
    d. NADH.

11. Which of the following defines *glycogenesis?*
    a. process of glycogen formation
    b. joining of glucose molecules
    c. catabolism of glycogen
    d. both a and b

12. Which of the following hormones helps glucose enter cells, and therefore decreases blood glucose?
    a. glucagon
    b. insulin
    c. epinephrine
    d. growth hormone

True or false

13. _____ Glycolysis is an anaerobic process.

14. _____ *Kilocalorie* and *calorie* are synonymous terms.

15. _____ Glycolysis occurs in the mitochondria, whereas the citric acid cycle occurs in the cytoplasm.

16. _____ Erythrocytes rely upon aerobic respiration.

17. _____ The process of gluconeogenesis synthesizes new glucose molecules.

18. _____ Glycogenesis is a homeostatic mechanism that functions when blood glucose levels increase above normal.

19. _____ Hyperglycemia occurs when the blood glucose dips below the normal set point level.

20. __T__ The conversion of proteins to glucose is an example of gluconeogenesis.

21. __T__ Glucagon stimulates glycogenolysis in the liver.

22. _____ ACTH decreases blood glucose concentration.

23. __F__ Disaccharides do *NOT* need to be chemically digested before they can be absorbed.

24. _____ The *citric acid cycle*, the *TCA cycle*, and the *Krebs cycle* are all synonymous.

25. _____ *Oxidative phosphorylation* refers to the joining of a phosphate group to ADP to form ATP.

26. _____ The breakdown of ATP molecules provides 50% of all of the energy that does cellular work.

27. _____ Glycogenolysis is consistent in all cells.

▷ *If you had difficulty with this section, review pages 996-1007.*

III—LIPIDS

Multiple Choice—select the best answer.

28. _____ contains fatty acid chains in which all available bonds of its hydrocarbon chain are filled with hydrogen atoms.
    a. Saturated fat
    b. Unsaturated fat
    c. Cholesterol
    d. both a and b

29. The most common lipids in the diet are:
    a. phospholipids.
    b. cholesterol.
    c. triglycerides.
    d. prostaglandins.

30. A high risk of atherosclerosis is associated with a high blood concentration of:
    a. LDL.
    b. HDL.
    c. CVA.
    d. both a and b.

31. All of the following hormones control lipid metabolism *EXCEPT*:
    a. ACTH.
    b. glucocorticoids.
    c. epinephrine.
    d. insulin.

32. Which of the following lab results would indicate high risk for atherosclerosis?
    a. 100 mg LDL/100 ml of blood
    b. 180 mg HDL/100 ml of blood
    c. 60 mg HDL/100 ml of blood
    d. 200 mg LDL/100 ml of blood

True or false

33. _____ A diet high in saturated fats and cholesterol tends to increase blood concentration of high-density lipoproteins.

34. _____ Lipid catabolism yields 9 kcal/g.

35. _____ Essential fatty acids are not synthesized by the body and must be obtained through the diet.

36. _____ Lipids are transported in the blood as chylomicrons, lipoproteins, and free fatty acids.

37. _____ The liver is the chief site of ketogenesis.

▷ *If you had difficulty with this section, review pages 1008-1011.*

IV—PROTEINS

Multiple Choice—select the best answer.

38. Which of the following is a nonessential amino acid?
    a. lysine
    b. alanine
    c. tryptophan
    d. valine

39. The process by which proteins are synthesized by the ribosomes in all cells is called:
    a. protein catabolism.
    b. protein anabolism.
    c. protein metabolism.
    d. both a and b.

40. Which of the following hormones tends to promote protein anabolism?
    a. testosterone
    b. growth hormone
    c. thyroid hormone
    d. all of the above

True or false

41. _____ In protein metabolism, catabolism is primary and anabolism is secondary.

42. _____ Foods from animal sources high in proteins contain the essential amino acids.

43. _____ Glucocorticoids are protein catabolic hormones.

44. _____ Growth and pregnancy usually result in a negative nitrogen balance.

45. _____ The first step in protein catabolism takes place in the liver and is called *deamination*.

V—VITAMINS AND MINERALS

Multiple Choice—select the best answer.

46. Which of the following plays an important role in detecting light in the sensory cells of the eye?
    a. vitamin D
    b. retinal
    c. biotin
    d. pantothenic acid

47. Which of the following vitamins is fat-soluble?
    a. vitamin A
    b. vitamin B
    c. vitamin C
    d. none of the above

48. Which of the following illnesses can result from an iodine deficiency?
    a. anemia
    b. bone degeneration
    c. goiter
    d. acid-base imbalance

True or false

49. _____ Athletic performance can be enhanced by vitamin supplementation.

50. _____ Vitamin E is thought to neutralize free radicals.

51. _____ Vitamin C deficiency could result in scurvy.

52. _____ Coenzymes are inorganic catalysts.

▷ *If you had difficulty with this section, review pages 1011-1018.*

VI—METABOLIC RATE AND MECHANISMS FOR REGULATING FOOD INTAKE

Multiple Choice—select the best answer.

53. Which of the following is *NOT* a condition required for the BMR?
    a. The individual is lying down and not moving.
    b. The individual is sleeping.
    c. It has been 12 to 18 hours since the individual's last meal.
    d. The individual is in a comfortable, warm environment.

54. Which of the following does *NOT* influence BMR?
    a. age
    b. gender
    c. ethnicity
    d. size

55. One pound of adipose tissue equals:
    a. 1000 kcal.
    b. 350 kcal.
    c. 3500 kcal.
    d. 10,000 kcal.

56. The appetite center is most likely located in the:
    a. cerebrum.
    b. hypothalamus.
    c. small intestine.
    d. stomach.

True or false

57. _____ Males have a BMR approximately 15–20% higher than females.

58. _____ Increases in blood temperature and glucose concentration may be linked to satiety.

59. _____ Body weight is linked to both energy input and energy output.

60. _____ When body temperature decreases, metabolism increases.

61. _____ Metabolic rate is the amount of energy released in the body in a given time by anabolism.

▷ *If you had difficulty with this section, review pages 1018-1023.*

VII—MECHANISMS OF DISEASE

Matching—choose the correct response.

a. phenylketonuria
b. anorexia nervosa
c. bulimia
d. obesity
e. PCM
f. marasmus
g. ascites

62. _____ characterized by a refusal to eat

63. _____ results from a deficiency of calories in general and protein in particular

64. _____ inborn error of metabolism

65. _____ advanced form of PCM

66. _____ not a disorder but may be a symptom of abnormal behavior

67. _____ binge-purge syndrome

68. _____ abdominal bloating

▷ *If you had difficulty with this section, review pages 1023-1026.*

Crossword Puzzle

Across
1. Decomposition process
4. Synthesis process
8. The food and nutrients we eat
9. Discovered citric acid cycle

Down
2. Does not require oxygen
3. Forms body fat from food
5. Requires oxygen
6. Chemical processes that make life possible
7. Organ molecule needed to assist enzyme functioning

APPLYING WHAT YOU KNOW

69. Dr. Reeder was concerned about Myrna. Her daily food intake provided fewer calories than her TMR. If this trend continues, what will be the result? If it continues over a long period of time, what eating disorder might Myrna develop?

70. Tom was experiencing fatigue and a blood test revealed that he was slightly anemic. What mineral(s) will his doctor most likely prescribe? What dietary sources might you suggest that he emphasize in his daily diet?

DID YOU KNOW ?

• The body's daily requirement of vitamins and minerals is less than a thimbleful.

• The average person consumes 2000 to 2500 calories a day but if you had the metabolism of a shrew you would need to consume approximately 200,000 calories a day! Smaller animals have higher metabolic rates because they have to work harder to keep their bodies warm.

ONE LAST QUICK CHECK

Multiple Choice—select the best answer.

71. What is the process by which pyruvic acid is broken down into carbon dioxide and high-energy electrons called?
    a. glycogenesis
    b. citric acid cycle
    c. glycolysis
    d. pyruvic acid cycle

72. The anabolism of glucose produces which of the following?
    a. glycogen
    b. amino acid
    c. rennin
    d. starch

73. Which of the following is a major hormone in the body that aids carbohydrate metabolism?
    a. oxytocin
    b. prolactin
    c. insulin
    d. ADH

74. The total metabolic rate is which of the following?
    a. the amount of fats we consume in a 24-hour period
    b. the same as the BMR
    c. the amount of energy expressed in calories used by the body per day
    d. cannot be calculated

75. When your consumption of calories equals your TMR, your weight will do which of the following?
    a. increase
    b. remain the same
    c. fluctuate
    d. decrease

76. What is the primary molecule the body usually breaks down as an energy source?
    a. amino acids
    b. pepsin
    c. maltose
    d. glucose

77. When glucose is *NOT* available, the body will next catabolize which of the following energy sources?
    a. fats
    b. proteins
    c. minerals
    d. vitamins

Circle the word or phrase that does not belong.

78. glycolysis	citric acid cycle	ATP	bile
79. adipose	amino acids	triglycerides	lipid
80. A	D	M	K
81. iron	protein	amino acids	essential
82. ACTH	insulin	growth hormone	epinephrine
83. sodium	calcium	zinc	folic acid
84. thiamine	niacin	ascorbic acid	riboflavin

Matching—identify the term that best matches the definition.

a. carbohydrate
b. fat
c. protein
d. vitamins
e. minerals

85. _____ preferred energy food

86. _____ amino acids

87. _____ fat-soluble

88. _____ required for nerve conduction

89. _____ glycolysis

90. _____ inorganic elements found naturally in the earth

91. _____ pyruvic acid

92. _____ chylomicrons

93. _____ triglycerides

CHAPTER 28

Urinary System

Living produces wastes. Wherever people live or work or play, wastes accumulate. To keep these areas healthy, there must be a method of disposing of these wastes such as a sanitation department.

Wastes also accumulate in your body. The conversion of food and gases into substances and energy necessary for survival results in waste products. A large percentage of these wastes is removed by the urinary system.

Two vital organs, the kidneys, cleanse the blood of the many waste products that are continually produced as a result of the metabolism of food in the body cells. They eliminate these wastes in the form of urine.

Urine formation is the result of three processes: filtration, reabsorption, and secretion. These processes occur in successive portions of the microscopic units of the kidneys known as *nephrons*. The amount of urine produced by the nephrons is controlled primarily by the hormones ADH and aldosterone. After the urine is produced, it is drained from the renal pelvis by the ureters to flow into the bladder. The bladder then stores the urine until it is voided through the urethra.

If waste products are allowed to accumulate in the body, they soon become poisonous, a condition called *uremia*. A knowledge of the urinary system is necessary to understand how the body rids itself of waste and avoids toxicity.

I—ANATOMY OF THE URINARY SYSTEM

Multiple Choice—select the best answer.

1. Which of the following is regulated by the kidneys?
   a. water content of the blood
   b. blood pH level
   c. blood ion concentration
   d. all of the above

2. The medial surface of each kidney has a notch called the:
   a. medulla.
   b. cortex.
   c. hilum.
   d. pelvis.

3. At the beginning of the "plumbing system" of the urinary system, urine leaving the renal papilla is collected in the cuplike structures called:
   a. renal columns.
   b. renal pyramids.
   c. calyces.
   d. ureters.

4. The functional unit of the kidney is the:
   a. renal corpuscle.
   b. nephron.
   c. juxtaglomerular apparatus.
   d. Bowman's capsule.

5. Which of the following is a component of the renal corpuscle?
   a. glomerulus
   b. Bowman's capsule
   c. afferent arteriole
   d. both a and b

6. Which of the following structures secretes renin when blood pressure in the afferent arteriole drops?
   a. renal tubule
   b. proximal convoluted tubule
   c. juxtaglomerular apparatus
   d. both a and b

7. Substances pass from the glomerulus and into the Bowman's capsule by:
   a. diffusion.
   b. active transport.
   c. filtration.
   d. osmosis.

8. The juxtaglomerular cells reside in the:
   a. afferent arteriole.
   b. efferent arteriole.
   c. proximal convoluted tubule.
   d. distal convoluted tubule.

True or false

9. _____ The left kidney is often slightly larger and positioned slightly lower than the right kidney.

10. _____ Blood is brought to the kidneys by the renal vein.

11. _____ *Micturition* and *urination* are synonymous terms.

12. _____ The glomerulus is one of the most important capillary networks for survival.

13. _____ Once urine enters the renal pelvis, it then travels to the renal calyces.

14. _____ As the basic functional unit of the kidney, the nephron's function is blood processing and urine formation.

15. _____ The kidneys are covered with visceral peritoneum.

Labeling—using the terms provided, label the following illustration of the kidney.

renal pelvis
renal papilla of pyramid
minor calyces
renal column
cortex

hilum
ureter
renal sinus
interlobular arteries

capsule (fibrous)
medulla
major calyces
medullary pyramid

Labeling—using the terms provided, label the following illustration of the nephron.

vasa recta
glomerulus
afferent arteriole
arcuate artery and vein
descending limb of Henle's loop
pyramid (medulla)
proximal tubule
efferent arteriole

interlobular vein and artery
ascending limb of Henle's loop
Henle's loop
collecting tubule
distal convoluted tubule
juxtamedullary nephron
cortical nephron

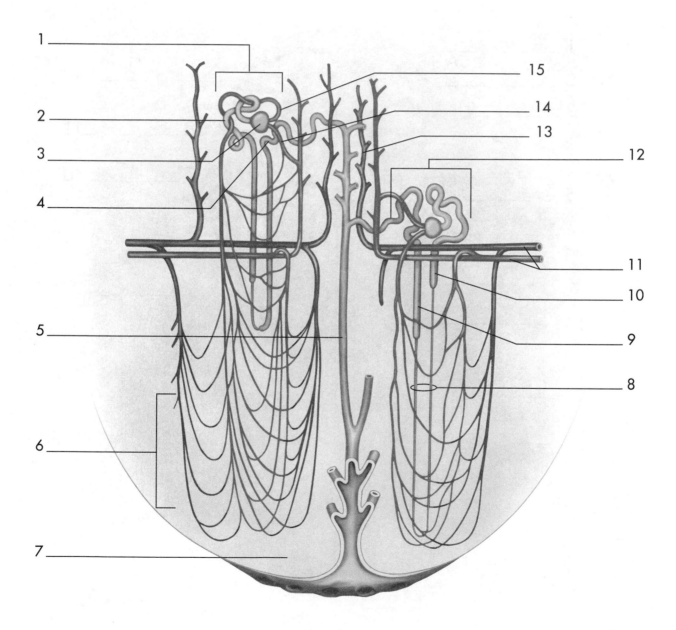

Labeling—label the following structure of the male urinary bladder.

▷ *If you had difficulty with this section, review pages 1034-1045.*

II—PHYSIOLOGY OF THE URINARY SYSTEM

Multiple Choice—select the best answer.

16. Which of the following is *NOT* one of the processes of urine formation?
    a. filtration
    b. diffusion
    c. reabsorption
    d. secretion

17. The movement of water and solutes from the plasma in the glomerulus, across the glomerular-capsular membrane, and into the capsular space of the Bowman's capsule, is termed:
    a. filtration.
    b. diffusion.
    c. reabsorption.
    d. secretion.

18. The movement of molecules out of the peritubular blood and into the tubule for excretion is:
    a. filtration.
    b. diffusion.
    c. reabsorption.
    d. secretion.

19. Under normal conditions, most water, electrolytes, and nutrients are reabsorbed in the:
    a. proximal convoluted tubule.
    b. distal convoluted tubule.
    c. loop of Henle.
    d. collecting duct.

20. Which of the following is considered a countercurrent structure?
    a. glomerulus
    b. proximal convoluted tubule
    c. loop of Henle
    d. distal convoluted tubule

21. Water loss from the blood is reduced by:
    a. ADH.
    b. ANH.
    c. aldosterone.
    d. both a and c.

22. *Dysuria* is a term describing:
    a. blood in the urine.
    b. pus in the urine.
    c. painful urination.
    d. absence of urine.

23. All of the following are normal contents of urine *EXCEPT*:
    a. nitrogenous wastes.
    b. hormones.
    c. pigments.
    d. plasma proteins.

24. Which of the following is *NOT* symptomatic of diabetes mellitus?
    a. copious urination
    b. glycosuria
    c. anuria
    d. diuresis

True or false

25. _____   Kidney failure means homeostatic failure, and if not relieved, inevitable death.

26. _____   Postexercise proteinuria is considered serious and often indicative of kidney disease.

27. _____   Fluid exiting the loop of Henle becomes less concentrated with Na$^+$ and Cl$^-$ ions.

28. _____   A hydrostatic pressure gradient drives the filtration out of the plasma and into the nephron.

29. _____   The efferent arteriole has a larger diameter than the afferent arteriole.

30. _____   Stress causes an increase in glomerular hydrostatic pressure.

31. _____   In the renal tubule, Na$^+$ is reabsorbed via active transport.

32. _____   Glomerular filtration separates only harmful substances from the blood.

33. _____   Urine consists of approximately 75% water.

34. _____   Urine has a pH of 4.6 to 8.0 and is generally alkaline.

35. _____   More than 99% of filtrates must be reabsorbed from the tubular segments of the nephron.

▷ *If you had difficulty with this section, review pages 1045-1057.*

III—MECHANISMS OF DISEASE

Matching—select the correct disorder from the choices provided.

a. pyelonephritis
b. renal colic
c. renal calculi
d. acute glomerulonephritis
e. proteinuria
f. uremia
g. neurogenic bladder
h. acute renal failure
i. hydronephrosis
j. chronic renal failure
k. cystitis
l. urethritis

36. _____   urine backs up into the kidneys causing swelling of the renal pelvis and calyces

37. _____   kidney stones

38. _____   final stage of chronic renal failure

39. _____   involuntary retention of urine with subsequent distention of the bladder

40. _____   inflammation of the bladder

41. _____   inflammation of the renal pelvis and connective tissues of the kidney

Matching—select the best answer to describe the terms.

a. involuntary voiding
b. passes through prostate gland
c. absence of urine
d. urination
e. blood in the urine
f. inflammation of the kidney
g. large amount of protein in urine
h. large amount of urine
i. folds that line the bladder
j. scanty amount of urine
k. test for renal dysfunction

60. _____ hematuria

61. _____ anuria

62. _____ nephritis

63. _____ micturition

64. _____ oliguria

65. _____ polyuria

66. _____ incontinence

67. _____ proteinuria

68. _____ rugae

69. _____ urethra

70. _____ BUN

CHAPTER 29

Fluid and Electrolyte Balance

Referring to the very first chapter in your text, you will recall that survival depends on the body's ability to maintain or restore homeostasis. Specifically, *homeostasis* means that the body fluids remain constant within very narrow limits. These fluids are classified as either intracellular fluid (ICF) or extracellular fluid (ECF). As their names imply, intracellular fluid lies within the cells and extracellular fluid is located outside the cells. A balance between these two fluids is maintained by several body mechanisms. Among them are: 1) the adjustment of fluid output to fluid intake under normal circumstances, 2) the concentration of electrolytes, 3) the capillary blood pressure, and 4) the concentration of proteins in the blood. Comprehension of how these mechanisms maintain and restore fluid balance is necessary for an understanding of the complexities of homeostasis and its relationship to the survival of the individual.

I—OVERVIEW OF FLUID AND ELECTROLYTE BALANCE

Multiple Choice—select the best answer.

1. The majority of total body water is found in the:
   a. plasma.
   b. interstitial fluid.
   c. intracellular fluid.
   d. extracellular fluid.

2. The most abundant intracellular cation is:
   a. Na^+.
   b. Cl^-.
   c. K^+.
   d. Mg^{++}.

3. The most abundant extracellular cation is:
   a. Na^+.
   b. Cl^-.
   c. K^+.
   d. Mg^{++}.

4. The most abundant anion in extracellular fluids is:
   a. Na^+.
   b. Cl^-.
   c. K^+.
   d. Mg^{++}.

5. Electrolyte reactivity is measured in:
   a. mg/100 L.
   b. milliequivalents.
   c. mEq/L.
   d. both b and c.

6. Which of the following mechanisms varies fluid output so that it equals input?
   a. antidiuretic device
   b. aldosterone mechanism
   c. renin-angiotensin mechanism
   d. both b and c

7. Which of the following is *NOT* one of the seven basic solutions used for parenteral therapy?
   a. ammonium chloride
   b. carbohydrate in water
   c. liquid protein
   d. Ringer's solution

True or false

8. _____ Obese people have a higher water content per kilogram of body weight than slender people.

9. _____ When compared chemically, plasma and interstitial fluid are nearly identical.

10. _____ Fluid intake usually equals fluid output.

11. _____ Electrolytes are substances that bind in water.

12. _____ Thirst is associated with any condition that decreases total volume of body water.

13. _____ Water exits the body only through the urinary and digestive systems.

14. _____ *Hypervolemia* refers to excess blood volume.

▷ *If you had difficulty with this section, review pages 1068-1074.*

II—MECHANISMS THAT MAINTAIN HOMEOSTASIS OF TOTAL FLUID VOLUME

Multiple Choice—select the best answer.

15. The two factors that determine urine volume are:
    a. the amount of ADH and aldosterone secretion.
    b. the amount of ACTH and ADH secretion.
    c. fluid intake and ADH secretion.
    d. the glomerular filtration rate and the rate of water reabsorption by the renal tubules.

16. Which of the following is an example of obligatory fluid output?
    a. water vapor in expired air
    b. water diffusion through the skin
    c. both a and b
    d. none of the above

True or false

17. _____ If a person takes nothing by mouth for several days, fluid output decreases to zero to compensate and maintain homeostasis.

18. _____ Dehydration is often detected by loss of skin elasticity.

▷ *If you had difficulty with this section, review pages 1074-1076.*

III—REGULATION OF WATER AND ELECTROLYTE LEVELS IN PLASMA, INTERSTITIAL FLUID, AND INTRACELLULAR FLUID

Multiple Choice—select the best answer.

19. Blood hydrostatic pressure:
    a. tends to force fluid out of capillaries and into interstitial fluid.
    b. tends to force fluid out of interstitial fluid and into capillaries.
    c. allows for an equilibrium across the capillary membrane.
    d. none of the above.

20. Which of the following is *NOT* a correct statement regarding severe dehydration?
    a. Loss of turgor is a symptom of severe dehydration.
    b. The relative loss of water in sweat is greater than the loss of electrolytes.
    c. Sweating serves the body by increasing body heat.
    d. Treatment of dehydration requires appropriate electrolyte replacement therapy.

21. The formula representing Starling's law of the capillaries is:
    a. (BHP + BCOP) − (IFCOP + IFHP) = EFP.
    b. (BHP + IFHP) − (IFCOP + BCOP) = EFP.
    c. (BHP + IFCOP) − (IFHP + BCOP) = EFP.

22. Which large molecules are retained by the selectively permeable cell membrane?
    a. sodium ions
    b. potassium ions
    c. proteins
    d. water

True or false

23. _____ *Edema* can be defined as "the presence of abnormally large amounts of fluid in the intercellular spaces of the body."

24. _____ The most common cause of edema is glomerulonephritis.

25. _____ The most significant player regulating intracellular fluid composition is the plasma membrane.

26. _____ Osmotic pressure is influenced by large protein molecules in the intracellular fluid.

▶ *If you had difficulty with this section, review pages 1076-1080.*

IV—REGULATION OF SODIUM AND POTASSIUM LEVELS IN BODY FLUIDS

True or false

27. _____ The release of ADH causes an increase in the reabsorption of sodium and water by the renal tubules.

28. _____ Over 8 liters of various internal secretions are produced daily.

29. _____ Potassium deficit is termed *hypokalemia*.

30. _____ Extracellular fluid depletion is said to be the "last line of defense" against dehydration.

31. _____ By volume, intestinal secretions are the largest sodium-containing internal secretions.

▶ *If you had difficulty with this section, review pages 1076 and 1080-1083.*

V—MECHANISMS OF DISEASE

Matching—identify the best answer for the terms.

a. dehydration
b. excessive perspiration
c. excess fluid volume
d. increased serum potassium
e. decreased serum sodium

32. _____ hypovolemia

33. _____ hyperkalemia

34. _____ hyponatremia

35. _____ diaphoresis

36. _____ hypervolemia

True or false

37. _____ Skin turgor is an important indicator of fluid volume stability.

38. _____ Cushing syndrome can cause hypokalemia.

39. _____ Overuse of diuretics can result in hyponatremia.

40. _____ Hyperkalemia is *NOT* a serious threat to the body.

▷ *If you had difficulty with this section, review pages 1083-1084.*

Crossword Puzzle

Across

1. Detect decreased blood pressure when dehydration occurs
4. Fluid volume excess
8. Fluid located within cells
9. Excessive loss of fluid from the body
10. Low serum potassium
11. Water found outside the cells

Down

2. Swelling
3. MEq
5. Fluid that surrounds the cells
6. Chloride deficiency
7. Administration of fluids by injection

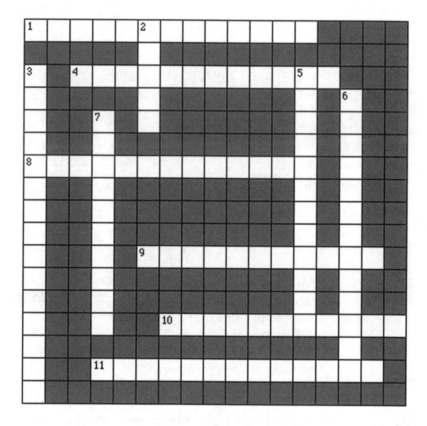

APPLYING WHAT YOU KNOW

41. Ms. Titus was asked to keep an accurate record of her fluid intake and output. She was concerned because the two did not balance, even though the physician assured her that she had no kidney pathology. What is a possible explanation for this?

42. Jack Sprat was 6' 5" and weighed 185 lbs. His wife was 5' 6" and weighed 185 lbs. Whose body contained more water?

DID YOU KNOW

- The best fluid replacement drink is to add 1/2 tsp of table salt to one quart of water.

- If all of the water were drained from the body of an average 160-pound man, the body would weigh 64 pounds.

ONE LAST QUICK CHECK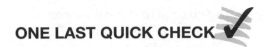

Circle the correct answer.

43. The largest volume of water by far lies (inside or outside) cells.

44. Interstitial fluid is (intracellular or extracellular).

45. Plasma is (intracellular or extracellular).

46. Obese people have a (lower or higher) water content per pound of body weight than thin people.

47. Infants have (more or less) water in comparison to body weight than adults of either sex.

48. In general, as age increases, the amount of water per pound of body weight (increases or decreases).

Multiple Choice—select the best answer.

49. Which one of the following is *NOT* a positively charged ion?
    a. chloride
    b. calcium
    c. sodium
    d. potassium

50. Which one of the following is *NOT* a negatively charged ion?
    a. chloride
    b. bicarbonate
    c. phosphate
    d. sodium

51. The smallest amount of water comes from:
    a. water in foods that are eaten.
    b. ingested food.
    c. water formed from catabolism.
    d. none of the above.

52. The greatest amount of water lost from the body is from the:
    a. lungs.
    b. skin by diffusion.
    c. skin by sweat.
    d. feces.
    e. kidneys.

53. Excessive water loss and fluid imbalance can result from which of the following?
    a. diarrhea
    b. vomiting
    c. severe burns
    d. all of the above

54. What factor is primarily responsible for moving water from interstitial fluid into blood?
    a. aldosterone secretions
    b. pressure in blood capillaries
    c. protein concentration of blood plasma
    d. antidiuretic hormone secretions

55. If blood sodium concentration decreases, what does blood volume do?
    a. increases
    b. decreases
    c. remains the same
    d. none of the above

56. Which of the following is true of body water?
    a. It is obtained from the liquids we drink.
    b. It is obtained from the foods we eat.
    c. It is formed by the catabolism of food.
    d. All of the above are true.

57. Edema may result from which of the following?
    a. retention of electrolytes
    b. decreased blood pressure
    c. increased concentration of blood plasma proteins
    d. all of the above

58. The most abundant and important positive plasma ion is which of the following?
    a. sodium
    b. chloride
    c. calcium
    d. oxygen

59. Which of the following is true when extracellular fluid volume decreases?
    a. aldosterone secretion increases
    b. kidney tubule reabsorption of sodium increases
    c. urine volume decreases
    d. all of the above are true

True or false

60. _____ Interstitial fluid contains hardly any protein anions.

61. _____ No net transfer of water occurs between blood and interstitial fluid as long as effective filtration (EFP) equals 0.

62. _____ Any change in the solute concentration of extracellular fluid will have a direct effect on water movement across the cell membrane in one direction or another.

CHAPTER 30

Acid-Base Balance

It has been established in previous chapters that an equilibrium between intracellular and extracellular fluid volume must exist for homeostasis. Equally important to homeostasis is the chemical acid-base balance of the body fluids. The degree of acidity or alkalinity of a body fluid is expressed in pH value. The neutral point, where a fluid would be neither acid nor alkaline, is pH 7. Increasing acidity is expressed as less than 7, and increasing alkalinity as greater than 7. Examples of body fluids that are acidic are gastric juice (1.6) and urine (6.0). Blood, on the other hand, is considered alkaline with a pH of 7.4.

Buffers are substances that prevent a sharp change in the pH of a fluid when an acid or base is added to it. They are one of several mechanisms that are constantly monitoring the pH of fluids in the body. If for any reason these mechanisms do not function properly, a pH imbalance occurs. These two kinds of imbalances are known as *alkalosis* and *acidosis*.

Maintaining the acid-base balance of body fluids is a matter of vital importance. If this balance varies even slightly, necessary chemical and cellular reactions cannot occur. Your review of this chapter is necessary to understand the delicate fluid balance necessary for survival.

I—MECHANISMS THAT CONTROL pH OF BODY FLUIDS

Multiple Choice—select the best answer.

1. As pH goes down, a:
   a. solution becomes more basic.
   b. solution's hydrogen ion concentration decreases.
   c. solution becomes more acidic.
   d. solution thickens.

2. The most acidic body substance of the following is:
   a. gastric juice.
   b. pancreatic juice.
   c. bile.
   d. urine.

3. Which of the following is an acid-forming food?
   a. grapefruit
   b. meat
   c. orange juice
   d. coffee

4. Which of the following is a base-forming food?
   a. fruit
   b. vegetable
   c. egg
   d. both a and b

5. Which of the following describes the narrow pH range of blood?
   a. 7.21 to 7.49
   b. 7.00 to 7.20
   c. 7.36 to 7.41
   d. 7.50 to 7.77

6. An acid-forming element is:
   a. sulfur.
   b. calcium.
   c. potassium.
   d. sodium.

7. Acidic ketone bodies are associated with cellular metabolism of:
   a. proteins.
   b. carbohydrates.
   c. fats.
   d. minerals.

True or false

8. _____ Blood is slightly alkaline.

9. _____ Citrus fruits, such as oranges and grapefruit, have a significant effect on acid-base balance.

10. _____ Chemical buffer systems are fast-acting.

11. _____ The carbon dioxide present in venous blood causes it to become slightly more basic than arterial blood.

12. _____ A vegetarian diet would tend to produce an alkaline state in body fluids.

13. _____ The respiratory and urinary systems can serve as physiological buffer systems.

▷ *If you had difficulty with this section, review pages 1090-1092.*

II—BUFFER MECHANISMS FOR CONTROLLING pH OF BODY FLUIDS

Multiple Choice—select the best answer.

14. Potassium salts of hemoglobin inside the red blood cell primarily buffer:
    a. carbonic acid.
    b. lactic acid.
    c. phosphoric acid.
    d. sulfuric acid.

15. A serious complication of vomiting is:
    a. carbonic acid. in blood
    b. bicarbonate deficit.
    c. metabolic alkalosis.
    d. metabolic acidosis.

True or false

16. _____ The process of exchanging a bicarbonate ion formed in the red blood cell with a chloride ion from the plasma is called *chloride shift.*

17. _F___ Buffers control pH in a manner that requires no other mechanism of pH control to maintain homeostasis.

18. _T___ The blood buffer system normally converts a strong acid to a weak acid.

19. _F___ Bicarbonate loading by athletes has proven to be mildly successful in diminishing the muscle soreness and fatigue associated with strenuous exercise.

20. _____ Elevated CO_2 levels result in increased formation of carbonic acid in red blood cells.

▷ *If you had difficulty with this section, review pages 1092-1095.*

III—RESPIRATORY AND URINARY MECHANISMS OF pH CONTROL

Multiple Choice—select the best answer.

21. With each expiration, which substances leave the body?
    a. CO_2
    b. H_2O
    c. O_2
    d. both a and b

22. All of the following would increase the respiration rate EXCEPT:
    a. decreased blood pH.
    b. decreased carbon dioxide.
    c. increased arterial blood CO_2.
    d. all increase respirations.

23. The kidney tubules secrete hydrogen ions in exchange of:
    a. K^+.
    b. Na^+.
    c. Ca^{++}.
    d. Cl^-.

24. Acidosis causes:
    a. hyperventilation.
    b. hypoventilation.
    c. an increase in blood pH.
    d. increase in potassium ion excretion.

25. A decrease in blood pH accelerates tubule excretion of:
    a. hydrogen.
    b. ammonia.
    c. both a and b.
    d. none of the above.

True or false

26. _____   Prolonged hyperventilation may increase blood pH enough to cause alkalosis.

27. _____   Respiratory mechanisms are much more effective in expelling hydrogen ions than are urinary mechanisms.

28. _____   The more hydrogen ions secreted by the renal tubule, the fewer potassium ions secreted.

29. _____   Intravenous administration of normal saline is used for metabolic acidosis.

30. _____   An increase in blood pH above normal (alkalosis) causes hypoventilation.

▷ *If you had difficulty with this section, review pages 1095-1098.*

IV—MECHANISMS OF DISEASE

Matching—write the letter of the correct term on the blank next to the appropriate definition.

a. metabolic acidosis
b. metabolic alkalosis
c. respiratory acidosis
d. respiratory alkalosis
e. treatment for metabolic and respiratory acidosis
f. uncompensated metabolic acidosis
g. hyperventilation

31. _____   result of untreated diabetes

32. _____   sodium lactate

33. _____   bicarbonate deficit

34. _____   bicarbonate excess

35. _____   rapid breathing

36. _____   carbonic acid excess

37. _____   carbonic acid deficit

▷ *If you had difficulty with this section, review pages 1100-1101.*

Crossword Puzzle

Across

3. May be caused by prolonged hypoventilation
4. pH greater than 7.0
6. Degree of acidity or alkalinity
7. Prevents swing in pH

Down

1. Complication of vomiting
2. Maintains electrical neutrality of red blood cells (two words)
5. pH less than 7.0

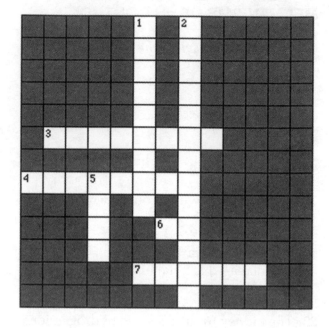

APPLYING WHAT YOU KNOW

38. Desi was pregnant and was experiencing repeated vomiting episodes for several days. Her doctor became concerned, admitted her to the hospital, and began intravenous administrations of normal saline. How will this help Desi?

39. Ginny had a minor bladder infection. She had heard that this is often the result of the urine being less acidic than necessary and that she should drink cranberry juice to correct the acid problem. She had no cranberry juice, so she decided to substitute orange juice. What was wrong with this substitution?

DID YOU KNOW

- English ships carried limes to protect the sailors from scurvy. American ships carried cranberries.

ONE LAST QUICK CHECK

Multiple Choice—select the best answer.

40. What happens as blood flows through lung capillaries?
    a. Carbonic acid in blood decreases.
    b. Hydrogen ions in blood decrease.
    c. Blood pH increases from venous to arterial blood.
    d. All of the above are true.

41. Which of the following organs is considered the most effective regulator of blood carbonic acid levels?
    a. kidneys
    b. intestines
    c. lungs
    d. stomach

42. Which of the following organs is considered the most effective regulator of blood pH?
    a. kidneys
    b. intestines
    c. lungs
    d. stomach

43. What is the pH of the blood?
    a. 7.0 to 8.0
    b. 7.6 to 7.8
    c. 6.2 to 7.4
    d. 7.3 to 7.4

44. If the ratio of sodium bicarbonate to carbonate ions is lowered (perhaps 10 to 1) and blood pH is also lowered, what is the condition called?
    a. uncompensated metabolic acidosis
    b. uncompensated metabolic alkalosis
    c. compensated metabolic acidosis
    d. compensated metabolic alkalosis

45. If a person hyperventilates for a given time period, which of the following will probably develop?
    a. metabolic acidosis
    b. metabolic alkalosis
    c. respiratory acidosis
    d. respiratory alkalosis

46. Which of the following is a characteristic of a buffer system in the body?
    a. It occurs in the case of prolonged vomiting.
    b. It results when the bicarbonate ion is present in excess.
    c. Therapy includes intravenous administration of normal saline.
    d. All of the above are true.

47. In the presence of a strong acid, which of the following is true?
    a. Sodium bicarbonate will react to produce carbonic acid.
    b. Sodium bicarbonate will react to produce more sodium bicarbonate.
    c. Carbonic acid will react to produce sodium bicarbonate.
    d. Carbonic acid will react to form more carbonic acid.

Matching—select the best answer for each item.

a. untreated diabetes mellitus
b. excessive vomiting
c. alkaline solution
d. "fixed" acid
e. barbiturate overdose
f. fever
g. acidic solution
h. prevent sharp pH changes

48. _____ pH lower than 7.0

49. _____ pH higher than 7.0

50. _____ buffers

51. _____ decrease in respirations

52. _____ increase in respirations

53. _____ metabolic acidosis

54. _____ metabolic alkalosis

55. _____ lactic acid

CHAPTER 31

Male Reproductive System

The reproductive system consists of those organs that participate in propagating the species. It is a unique body system in that its organs differ between the two sexes, and yet the goal of creating a new being is the same. Of interest also is the fact that this system is the only one not necessary to the survival of the individual, and yet survival of the species depends on the proper functioning of the reproductive organs. The male reproductive system is divided into the external genitals, testes, duct system, and accessory glands. The testes, or gonads, are considered essential organs because they produce the sex cells—sperm—which join with the female sex cells—ova—to form a new human being. They also secrete testosterone, the male sex hormone, which is responsible for the physical transformation of a boy to a man.

Sperm are formed in the testes by the seminiferous tubules. From there they enter a long narrow duct, the epididymis. They continue onward through the vas deferens into the ejaculatory duct, down the urethra, and out of the body. Throughout this journey, various glands secrete substances that add motility to the sperm and create a chemical environment conducive to reproduction.

A knowledge of the male reproductive system is necessary to understand the role of the male and the phenomena necessary to produce an offspring.

I—MALE REPRODUCTIVE ORGANS

Multiple Choice—select the best answer.

1. The male gonads are known as the:
   a. testes.
   b. prostate.
   c. epididymis.
   d. perineum.

2. The region within a "triangle" created by the ischial tuberosities and the symphysis is the:
   a. anal triangle.
   b. urogenital triangle.
   c. perineal triangle.
   d. testicular triangle.

3. Which of the following is *NOT* a supporting structure?
   a. penis
   b. scrotum
   c. prostate
   d. spermatic cord

4. Each testicular lobule contains:
   a. seminiferous tubules.
   b. interstitial cells.
   c. Leydig cells.
   d. all of the above.

5. The blood-testis barrier is formed by tight junctions between which cells?
   a. Leydig cells
   b. interstitial cells
   c. Sertoli cells
   d. all of the above

6. Sperm production occurs in the:
   a. seminiferous tubules.
   b. interstitial cells.
   c. Sertoli cells.
   d. prostate.

7. Which hormone is responsible for the stimulation of sperm production?
   a. FSH
   b. LH
   c. testosterone
   d. both b and c

8. Which of the following is *NOT* a specific region of a spermatozoon?
   a. head
   b. middle piece
   c. body
   d. tail

True or false

9. _____ The testes perform two primary functions: spermatogenesis and secretion of hormones.

10. _____ Testosterone is secreted by the anterior pituitary.

11. _____ Testicular cancer is the most common neoplasm in elderly men.

12. _____ *Capacitation* refers to the release of enzymes contained within the acrosome.

13. _____ *Sertoli cells* and *efferent ductules* are synonymous.

14. _____ The bulbourethral glands are a supporting structure of the male reproductive system.

15. _____ Testosterone is sometimes referred to as "the anabolic hormone."

Labeling—label the following sagittal section of the pelvis depicting placement of male reproductive organs.

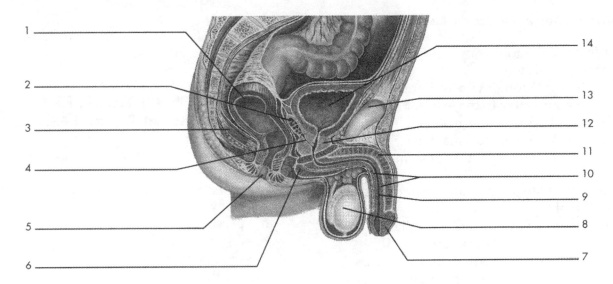

Labeling—using the terms provided, label the following tubules of the testis and epididymis.

seminiferous tubules
tunica albuguinea
epididymis
lobule

septum
spermatic cord (nerves and blood vessels)
ductus deferens (vas)
testis

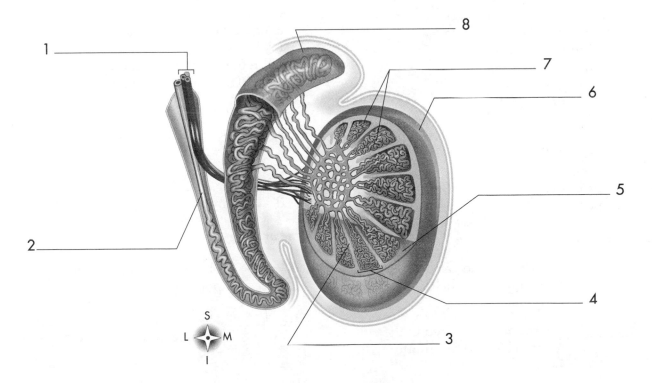

▷ *If you had difficulty with this section, review pages 1110-1115.*

II—REPRODUCTIVE DUCTS AND ACCESSORY REPRODUCTIVE GLANDS

Multiple Choice—select the best answer.

16. Which of the following is *NOT* a function of the epididymis?
    a. a duct through which sperm travel on their journey to the exterior of the body
    b. production of spermatozoa
    c. maturation of spermatozoa
    d. secretion of a portion of seminal fluid

17. The ejaculatory ducts are formed by the union of the:
    a. seminal vesicles and ampulla.
    b. vas deferens and urethra.
    c. seminal vesicles and vas deferens.
    d. seminal vesicles and urethra.

18. Which of the following accessory reproductive glands produce(s) a secretion rich in fructose?
    a. seminal vesicles
    b. prostate
    c. bulbourethral gland
    d. Cowper's gland

19. Which of the following accessory glands secrete(s) an alkaline substance?
    a. seminal vesicles
    b. bulbourethral gland
    c. all of the above
    d. none of the above

20. The most common cancer in American men is cancer of the:
    a. testes.
    b. prostate.
    c. penis.

True or false

21. _____ The duct of the vas deferens is an extension of the tail of the epididymis.

22. _____ Sperm may be stored in the epididymis for up to a month with no loss of fertility.

23. _____ A vasectomy is a procedure intended to render a man sterile.

24. _____ Prostate-specific antigen (PSA) is present in the blood of men with prostate cancer.

▶ *If you had difficulty with this section, review pages 1116-1120.*

III—SUPPORTING STRUCTURES, SEMINAL FLUID, AND MALE FERTILITY

Multiple Choice—select the best answer.

25. The greatest amount of seminal fluid is secreted by the:
    a. prostate.
    b. testes.
    c. seminal vesicles.
    d. epididymis.

26. Elevation of the testes is caused by contraction of the:
    a. dartos fascia and muscle.
    b. cremaster muscle.
    c. corpora cavernosa.
    d. corpus spongiosum.

27. Functional sterility results when sperm count falls below:
    a. 5 million/ml of semen.
    b. 25 million/ml of semen.
    c. 100 million/ml of semen.
    d. 500 million/ml of semen.

28. Which of the following factors related to sperm does *NOT* affect male fertility?
    a. size
    b. shape
    c. texture
    d. motility

True or false

29. _____ The urethra lies within the corpora cavernosa.

30. _____ The terminal end of the corpus spongiosum forms the glans penis.

31. _____ *Emission* and *ejaculation* are synonymous terms.

Labeling—using the terms provided, label the following parts of the penis.

corpus cavernosum   urethra
bulb   crus penis
glans penis   corpus spongiosum
bulbourethral gland   foreskin (prepuce)
deep artery   external urethral orifice
openings of ejaculatory ducts   bladder
prostate   opening of Cowper's glands

▷ *If you had difficulty with this section, review pages 1120-1122.*

IV—MECHANISMS OF DISEASE

Fill in the blanks.

32. Decreased sperm production is called
    _____.

33. Testes normally descend into the scrotum
    about _____ before birth.

34. If a baby is born with undescended testes,
    a condition called _____
    results.

35. A common noncancerous condition of the
    prostate in older men is known as

    _____ _____
    _____.

36. _____ is a condition in
    which the foreskin fits so tightly over the
    glans that it cannot retract.

37. Failure to achieve an erection of the penis is
    called _____ or _____
    _____.

38. An accumulation of fluid in the scrotum is
    known as a _____.

39. An _____

_____ results when the intestines push through the weak area of the abdominal wall that separates the abdominopelvic cavity from the scrotum.

▷ *If you had difficulty with this section, review pages 1122-1124.*

Crossword Puzzle

Across

4. Male organ of copulation
5. Accessory reproductive gland
7. Provide protection for germ cells (two words)
8. Sex cell
10. Ejaculate from the penis
11. Male sex hormone
12. Reproductive organs

Down

1. Sex glands where reproductive cells are formed
2. Androgen
3. Genital duct
6. Mature male gametes
9. Male gonads

APPLYING WHAT YOU KNOW

40. Trent is an infant who was born with undescended testes. What is the clinical term for his condition? How easily is this diagnosed? What can Trent's doctor do to treat his condition? How serious is his condition if left untreated? What are his chances of normal testicular and sexual development?

41. John noticed an unusual swelling of his scrotum. What possible conditions may he be experiencing? Also, he did notice that the swelling occurred after a day of heavy lifting while moving out of his apartment. Based on this detail, which condition is he more likely to be experiencing? Describe the anatomy of this condition. How will the doctor treat John?

DID YOU KNOW?

- The testes produce approximately 50 million sperm per day. Every 2 to 3 months they produce enough cells to populate the entire earth.

- Men reach the peak of their sexual powers in their late teens or early twenties, and then begin to slowly decline. Women however, do not reach their sexual peak until their late twenties or early thirties, and then remain at this level through their late fifties or early sixties.

ONE LAST QUICK CHECK ✔

Multiple Choice—select the best answer.

42. The testes are suspended outside the body cavity to do which of the following?
    a. protect them from trauma
    b. keep them cooler
    c. keep them supplied with a greater number of blood vessels
    d. protect them from infection

43. What is the removal of the foreskin from the glans penis called?
    a. vasectomy
    b. sterilization
    c. circumcision
    d. ligation

44. The testes are surrounded by a tough membrane called the:
    a. ductus deferens.
    b. tunica albuginea.
    c. septum.
    d. seminiferous membrane

45. The _____ lie near the septa that separate the lobules.
    a. ductus deferens
    b. sperm
    c. interstitial cells
    d. nerves

46. Sperm are found in the walls of the:
    a. seminiferous tubule.
    b. interstitial cells.
    c. septum.
    d. blood vessels.

47. The scrotum provides an environment that is approximately _____ for the testes.
    a. the same as the body temperature
    b. 5° warmer than the body temperature
    c. 3° warmer than the body temperature
    d. 3° cooler than the body temperature

48. The _____ produce(s) testosterone.
    a. seminiferous tubules
    b. prostate gland
    c. bulbourethral glands
    d. interstitial cells

49. The part of the sperm that contains genetic information that will be inherited is the:
    a. tail.
    b. acrosome.
    c. middle piece.
    d. head.

50. Which one of the following is *NOT* a function of testosterone?
    a. It causes a deepening of the voice.
    b. It promotes the development of the male accessory organs.
    c. It has a stimulatory effect on protein catabolism.
    d. It causes greater muscular development and strength.

51. Sperm production is called:
    a. spermatogonia.
    b. spermatids.
    c. spermatogenesis.
    d. spermatocyte.

52. The section of the sperm that contains enzymes that enable it to break down the covering of the ovum and permit entry should contact occur is the:
    a. acrosome.
    b. middle piece.
    c. tail.
    d. stem.

Matching—insert the letter in the space next to the appropriate description.

a. epididymis
b. vas deferens
c. ejaculatory duct
d. prepuce
e. seminal vesicles
f. prostate gland
g. Cowper's gland
h. corpus spongiosum
i. semen
j. spermatic cord

53. _____ continuation of ducts that start in the epididymis

54. _____ erectile tissue

55. _____ also known as *bulbourethral*

56. _____ narrow tube that lies along the top of and behind the testes

57. _____ doughnut-shaped gland beneath the bladder

58. _____ union of the vas deferens with the ducts from the seminal vesicles

59. _____ mixture of sperm and secretions of accessory sex glands

60. _____ contributes 60% of the seminal fluid volume

61. _____ removed during circumcision

62. _____ enclose the vas deferens, blood vessels, lymphatics, and nerves

CHAPTER 32

Female Reproductive System

The female reproductive system is truly extraordinary and diverse. It produces ova, receives the penis and sperm during intercourse, is the site of conception, houses and nourishes the embryo during the prenatal development, and nourishes the infant after birth.

Because of its diversity, the physiology of the female is generally considered to be more complex than that of the male. Much of the activity of this system revolves around the menstrual cycle and the monthly preparation that the female undergoes for a possible pregnancy.

The organs of this system are divided into essential organs and accessory organs of reproduction. The essential organs of the female are the ovaries. Just as with the male, the essential organs of the female are referred to as the *gonads*. The gonads of the female produce ova and are responsible for producing hormones necessary for the appearance of the secondary sex characteristics.

The menstrual cycle of the female typically covers a period of 28 days. Each cycle consists of three phases: menstrual period, postmenstrual phase, and premenstrual phase. Changes in the blood levels of the hormones that are responsible for the menstrual cycle also cause physical and emotional changes in the female. A knowledge of these phenomena and the female system are necessary to complete your understanding of the reproductive system.

I—OVERVIEW OF THE FEMALE REPRODUCTIVE SYSTEM

Multiple Choice—select the best answer.

1. Which of the following is *NOT* an accessory organ of reproduction in women?
   a. ovaries
   b. uterus
   c. vagina
   d. vulva

2. The term that refers to the external female genitalia is:
   a. vagina.
   b. vulva.
   c. perineum.
   d. urogenital triangle.

True or false

3. _____ Mammary glands are referred to as *additional sex glands*.

4. _____ An episiotomy is associated with the perineum.

Labeling—match each term with its corresponding number in the following frontal section of the female pelvic organs.

fundus of uterus

cervical canal

vagina

endometrium

cervix of uterus

myometrium

fallopian tube (uterine tube)

body of uterus

fimbriae

follicle

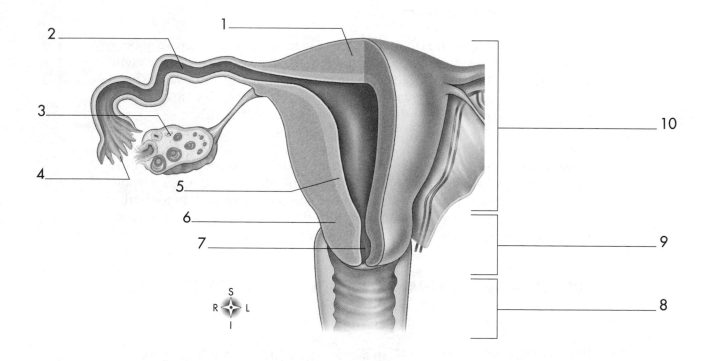

Labeling—label the following sagittal section of the pelvis showing the female reproductive organs.

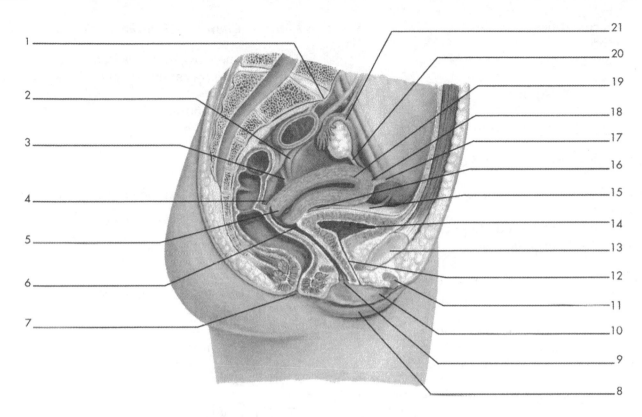

▷ *If you had difficulty with this section, review page 1130.*

II—INTERNAL FEMALE GENITALS

Multiple Choice—select the best answer.

5. The ovaries are homologous to the male:
    a. prostate.
    b. testes.
    c. vas deferens.
    d. seminal vesicle.

6. Cells of ovarian tissue secrete:
    a. estradiol.
    b. estrone.
    c. progesterone.
    d. all of the above.

7. The bulging upper component of the uterus is the:
    a. cervix.
    b. fundus.
    c. body.
    d. fornix.

8. The innermost lining of the uterus is the:
    a. endometrium.
    b. myometrium.
    c. perimetrium.
    d. parietal peritoneum.

9. The portion of the uterus that opens into the vagina is the:
    a. internal os.
    b. external os.
    c. fornix.
    d. cervix.

10. The fringelike projections of the uterine tubes are called the:
    a. isthmus.
    b. ampulla.
    c. infundibulum.
    d. fimbriae.

Matching—insert the letter of the correct structure in the blank next to the description.

a. uterine tubes
b. uterus
c. vagina

11. _____ isthmus

12. _____ myometrium

13. _____ terminal end of birth canal

14. _____ site of menstruation

15. _____ intermediate portion called the *ampulla*

16. _____ consists of body, fundus, and cervix

17. _____ site of fertilization

18. _____ also known as *oviduct*

19. _____ receptacle for sperm

True or false

20. _____ Ovarian follicles contain oocytes.

21. _____ *Retroflexion* refers to the normal position of the uterus in relation to the vagina and urinary bladder.

22. _____ The afterbirth is also referred to as the *fornix*.

23. _____ The "G spot" is an "erotic zone" described by Dr. Grafenberg.

▷ *If you had difficulty with this section, review page 1130-1138.*

III—EXTERNAL FEMALE GENITALS AND BREASTS

Multiple Choice—select the best answer.

24. The female organ that is homologous to the male corpora cavernosa and glans penis is the:
    a. labia minora.
    b. labia majora.
    c. clitoris.
    d. vulva.

25. The area between the labia minora is the:
    a. vulva.
    b. vestibule.
    c. mons pubis.
    d. "G spot."

26. Which of the following is *NOT* a structure of the vulva?
    a. vagina
    b. labia majora
    c. urinary meatus
    d. clitoris

27. Which of the following hormones are *NOT* involved with lactation?
    a. thyroxin
    b. oxytocin
    c. estrogen
    d. progesterone

True or false

28. _____ The mons pubis serves as a boundary between the external and internal female genitals.

29. _____ The larger the breasts, the greater amount of glandular tissue present.

30. _____ Milk secretion from the breasts begins about 3 or 4 hours after giving birth.

31. _____ Milk ejection is stimulated by oxytocin.

32. _____ Human milk provides active immunity to the offspring in the form of maternal antibodies.

▷ *If you had difficulty with this section, review page 1138-1141.*

IV—FEMALE REPRODUCTIVE CYCLE

Multiple Choice—select the best answer.

33. Menses occurs on days _____ of a new cycle.
    a. 1 to 5
    b. 1 to 14
    c. 6 to 14
    d. none of the above

34. Ovulation usually occurs on cycle day _____ of a 28-day cycle.
    a. 1
    b. 7
    c. 14
    d. 28

35. Failure to have a menstrual cycle is termed:
    a. infertility.
    b. menarche.
    c. menses.
    d. amenorrhea.

36. Which of the following hormones triggers ovulation?
    a. estrogen
    b. progesterone
    c. luteinizing hormone
    d. follicle-stimulating hormone

37. The average age at which menopause occurs is:
    a. 40 years.
    b. 45 to 50 years.
    c. 55 to 60 years.
    d. 60 to 65 years.

True or false

38. _____ The time of ovulation can be easily predicted by simply knowing the length of a previous cycle.

39. _____ Cyclical changes in the ovaries result from cyclical changes in the amounts of gonadotropins secreted by the anterior pituitary.

40. _____ Contraceptive pills and implants function by preventing ovulation.

41. _____ The first menstrual flow is known as the *climacteric*.

42. _____ The LH surge occurs at the beginning of the menstrual cycle.

▷ *If you had difficulty with this section, review page 1141-1148.*

V—MECHANISMS OF DISEASE

Matching—choose the correct response.

a. amenorrhea
b. dysmenorrhea
c. exogenous infection
d. DUB
e. myoma
f. vaginitis
g. sexually transmitted disease (STD)
h. Candidiasis
i. scabies
j. Pap smear
k. genital herpes
l. Trichomoniasis

43. _____ often occurs from STDs or from a "yeast infection"

44. _____ benign tumor of smooth muscle and fibrous connective tissue; also known as a *fibroid tumor*

45. _____ absence of normal menstruation

46. _____ yeast infection characterized by leukorrhea

47. _____ caused by infestation by the itch mite

48. _____ venereal disease

49. _____ results from pathogenic organisms transmitted from another person; e.g., STD

50. _____ painful menstruation

51. _____ asymptomatic in most women and nearly all men

52. _____ results from a hormonal imbalance rather than from an infection or disease condition

53. _____ screening test for cervical cancer

54. _____ causes blisters on the skin of the genitals; the blisters may disappear temporarily, but recur, especially as a result of stress

▷ *If you had difficulty with this section, review page 1149-1154.*

Crossword Puzzle

Across
5. Female sex hormone
6. Release of ovum
9. Secretion of milk
11. Climacteric

Down
1. Fallopian tube (two words)
2. Menarche
3. Lower portion of birth canal
4. Lining of uterus
7. External genitalia
8. Womb
10. Female gonad

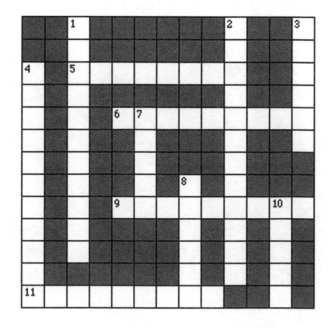

APPLYING WHAT YOU KNOW

55. Prior to having children, Lorena used oral contraceptives to prevent an unwanted pregnancy with her husband. Describe the physiological mechanism of action of oral contraceptives. After having three children by the age of 35, the couple decided that Lorena would have a tubal ligation. Describe how this procedure prevents pregnancy.

56. Mary contracted gonorrhea. By the time she made an appointment to see her doctor, it had spread to her abdominal organs. How is this possible when gonorrhea is a disease of the reproductive system?

DID YOU KNOW?

- During menstruation, the sensitivity of a woman's middle finger is reduced.

- During pregnancy, the uterus expands to 500 times its normal size.

- There are an estimated 925,000 daily occurrences of STD transmission and 550,000 daily pregnancies worldwide.

ONE LAST QUICK CHECK

Matching—select the best answer for the descriptions.

a. salpingitis
b. vulva
c. mittelschmerz
d. colostrum
e. ectopic
f. G spot
g. ovary
h. endometriosis
i. climacteric
j. gestation

57. _____ essential organ of reproduction

58. _____ external reproductive organ

59. _____ pregnancy in a location other than the uterus

60. _____ term of pregnancy

61. _____ inflammation of the uterine tube

62. _____ erotic zone

63. _____ middle pain

64. _____ menopause

65. _____ displaced endometrial tissue

66. _____ thin, yellow secretion

Fill in the blanks.

67. The _____ _____ phase occurs between ovulation and the onset of the menses.

68. _____ stimulates breast alveoli to secrete milk.

69. _____ stimulates breast alveoli to eject milk.

70. Sexual cell division is known as _____.

71. Immediately after ovulation, cells of the ruptured follicle enlarge and become transformed into the _____ _____.

72. _____ measures blood levels of gonadotropins.

73. _____ is marked by the passage of one full year without menstruation.

74. _____ are the most common of all communicable diseases.

75. _____ uterine ligaments hold the uterus in its normal position by anchoring it in the pelvic cavity.

76. The _____ permits exchange of materials between the offspring's blood and the maternal blood.

CHAPTER 33

Growth and Development

Millions of fragile microscopic sperm swim against numerous obstacles to reach the ova and create a new life. At birth, the newborn will fill his lungs with air and cry lustily, signaling to the world that he is ready to begin the cycle of life. This cycle will be marked by ongoing changes, periodic physical growth, and continuous development.

This chapter reviews the more significant events that occur in the normal growth and development of an individual from conception to death. Realizing that each person is unique, we nonetheless can discover amid all the complexities of humanity some constants that are understandable and predictable.

A knowledge of human growth and development is essential in understanding the commonalties that influence individuals as they pass through the cycle of life.

I—A NEW HUMAN LIFE

Multiple Choice—select the best answer.

1. Which of the following processes reduces the number of chromosomes in each daughter cell to half the number present in the parent cell?
   a. mitosis
   b. meiosis
   c. prophase
   d. telophase

2. Forty-six chromosomes per body cell is known as the _____ number of chromosomes.
   a. haploid
   b. diploid
   c. tetrad
   d. both a and c

3. Each primary spermatocyte undergoes meiotic division I to form:
   a. four haploid secondary spermatocytes.
   b. four diploid secondary spermatocytes.
   c. one diploid secondary spermatocyte.
   d. two haploid secondary spermatocytes.

4. A mature follicle ready to burst open from the ovary's surface is a:
    a. graafian follicle.
    b. theca cell.
    c. zygote.
    d. first polar body.

5. Fertilization occurs in the:
    a. ovary.
    b. fallopian tubes.
    c. uterus.
    d. vagina.

6. The phenomenon of "crossing over" takes place during:
    a. meiosis I only.
    b. meiosis II only.
    c. both meiosis I and meiosis II.
    d. both meiosis and mitosis.

True or false

7. _____   Sex cells contain 23 chromosomes and are therefore referred to as *diploid*.

8. _____   The process of "crossing over" allows for almost infinite variety to the genetic makeup of an individual.

9. _____   Completion of meiosis II in the released oocyte requires the head of a sperm cell to enter the oocyte.

10. _____   *Zygote* is the term used to describe the ovulated ovum that is awaiting fertilization.

11. _____   *Insemination* and *fertilization* are synonymous terms.

12. _____   The ovum can live for up to 3 days.

13. _____   During oogenesis, the cytoplasm is not equally divided among daughter cells.

14. _____   Sperm cells can live in the female reproductive tract for up to 3 days.

▶ *If you had difficulty with this section, review pages 1162-1169.*

II—PRENATAL PERIOD

Multiple Choice—select the best answer.

15. About 3 days after fertilization, the zygote forms into a solid mass of cells called a:
    a. morula.
    b. blastocyst.
    c. inner cell mass.
    d. embryo.

16. The outer wall of the blastocyst is referred to as the:
    a. yolk sac.
    b. trophoblast.
    c. chorion.
    d. morula.

17. The "bag of waters" is also called the:
    a. amniotic sac.
    b. yolk sac.
    c. chorion.
    d. placenta.

18. Which of the following is *NOT* a primary germ layer?
    a. ectoderm
    b. exoderm
    c. endoderm
    d. mesoderm

19. By which month of fetal development are all organ systems formed and functioning?
    a. second
    b. third
    c. fourth
    d. fifth

True or false

20. __T__   Placental tissue secretes large amounts of human chorionic gonadotropin (HCG) early in pregnancy.

21. __F__   The yolk sac plays a critical role in the nutrition of the developing human offspring.

22. _____   The process by which the primary germ layers develop into many different kinds of tissues is called *organogenesis*.

23. _____   The blastocyst is a hollow ball of cells.

24. _____   Division of the cells of the zygote is called *cleavage*.

▷ *If you had difficulty with this section, review pages 1169-1181.*

III—BIRTH, OR PARTURITION, AND THE POSTNATAL PERIOD

Multiple Choice—select the best answer.

25. Stage two of labor is best described as the:
    a. onset of contractions until uterine dilation is complete.
    b. expulsion of the placenta through the vagina.
    c. time of maximum cervical dilation until the baby exits through the vagina.
    d. time after the baby exits through the vagina and the cervix regains normal aperture.

26. Fraternal twins:
    a. are also called *identical twins*.
    b. arise from the same zygote.
    c. arise from two different sperm and two different ova.
    d. arise from a single sperm.

27. The period of infancy lasts approximately from birth to:
    a. 4 weeks.
    b. 6 months.
    c. 12 months.
    d. 18 months.

28. A rare, inherited condition in which an individual appears to age rapidly is:
    a. senescence.
    b. progeria.
    c. preeclampsia.
    d. teratogenia.

29. Birth weight generally triples by:
    a. 6 months.
    b. 12 months.
    c. 18 months.
    d. 24 months.

True or false

30. _____   A cesarean section is a surgical procedure that delivers a newborn through an incision in the abdomen and uterine wall.

31. _____   When a single zygote divides early in its development and forms two separate individuals, it is referred to as *identical twinning*.

32. _____   Stage one of labor usually lasts from a few minutes to an hour.

33. _____   Neonates have both a lumbar and thoracic curve to their spines.

34. _____   Girls experience adolescent growth spurt before boys do.

▷ *If you had difficulty with this section, review pages 1181-1187.*

IV—EFFECTS OF AGING

Multiple Choice—select the best answer.

35. A sound exercise program throughout life could reduce the effects of aging in which of the following body systems?
    a. cardiovascular
    b. skeletal
    c. muscular
    d. all of the above

36. Clouding of the lens of the eye is called:
    a. presbyopia.
    b. myopia.
    c. glaucoma.
    d. cataract.

True or false

37. _____   The number of functioning nephron units in the kidneys decreases by almost 50% between the ages of 30 and 75.

38. _____   Progesterone therapy may be used to relieve some symptoms of menopause.

▷ *If you had difficulty with this section, review pages 1187-1191.*

V—MECHANISMS OF DISEASE

Matching—select the best answer for the descriptions.

a. placenta previa
b. tubal pregnancy
c. preeclampsia
d. spontaneous abortion
e. stillbirth
f. birth defects
g. puerperal fever
h. mastitis
i. teratogens
j. abruptio placentae

39. _____ pregnancy-induced hypertension

40. _____ placenta grows too close to the cervical opening

41. _____ miscarriage

42. _____ common type of ectopic pregnancy

43. _____ breast inflammation

44. _____ congenital abnormalities

45. _____ separation of placenta from uterine wall

46. _____ childbed fever

▷ *If you had difficulty with this section, review pages 1191-1192.*

Crossword Puzzle

Across
6. Study of individual development before birth
9. Hollow ball that implants itself in the uterus
10. Conception
11. Birth
12. Process where germ layers develop into various tissues

Down
1. Solid mass formed by zygote
2. First 4 weeks of infancy
3. Fertilized ovum
4. Attachment of fertilized ovum in uterus
5. Older adulthood
7. Length of pregnancy
8. Develops from the trophoblast

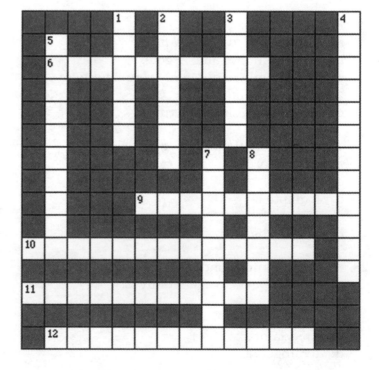

APPLYING WHAT YOU KNOW

47. John is 70 years old. He has always enjoyed food and has a hearty appetite. Lately, however, he has complained that food "just doesn't taste as good anymore." What might be a possible explanation?

48. Gary and Harry were identical twins. Christine gave birth to a baby boy and identified Gary as the father of the child on the birth certificate. Paternity testing later revealed that both twins were the father. How is this possible?

DID YOU KNOW ?

• A 3-week-old embryo is no larger than a sesame seed. A 1-month-old fetus's body is no heavier than an envelope and a sheet of paper. Its hand is no bigger than a teardrop.

• Between the ages of 30 and 70, a nose may lengthen and widen by as much as half an inch and the ears may be a quarter-inch longer because cartilage is one of the few tissues that continues to grow as we age.

ONE LAST QUICK CHECK

Matching—choose the correct term for the appropriate description.

a. laparoscope
b. gestation
c. antenatal
d. histogenesis
e. C-section
f. endoderm
g. in vitro
h. parturition
i. embryonic phase
j. ultrasonogram

49. _____   "within a glass"

50. _____   inside germ layer

51. _____   before birth

52. _____   length of pregnancy

53. _____   fiberoptic viewing instrument

54. _____   process of birth

55. _____   surgical procedure in which a newborn is delivered through an incision in the abdomen and uterine wall

56. _____   study of how the primary germ layers develop into many different kinds of tissues

57. _____   fertilization until the end of the eighth week of gestation

58. _____   monitors progress of developing fetus.

Multiple Choice—select the best answer.

59. Degenerative changes in the urinary system that accompany old age include which of the following?
    a. decreased capacity of the bladder and the inability to empty or void completely
    b. decrease in the number of nephrons
    c. less blood flow through the kidneys

60. Any hardening of the arteries is referred to as which of the following?
    a. angioma
    b. atherosclerosis
    c. angina
    d. arteriosclerosis
    e. all of the above

61. Which of the following is characteristic of the disorder called *presbyopia*?
    a. It is very characteristic of old age.
    b. If causes farsightedness in some individuals.
    c. It is characterized by a lens in the eye becoming hard and losing its elasticity.
    d. All of the above are true.

62. Which of the following events, if any, is *NOT* characteristic of adolescence?
    a. bone closure occurs
    b. secondary sexual characteristics develop
    c. very rapid growth occurs
    d. all of the above events are characteristic of adolescence

63. Which of the following structures is derived from ectoderm?
    a. lining of the lungs
    b. brain
    c. kidneys
    d. all of the above

Matching—select the best answer from the list of descriptions.

a. older adulthood
b. study of aging
c. Hutchinson-Gilford disease
d. fat accumulation in arteries
e. secondary sexual characteristics

64. _____ atherosclerosis

65. _____ adolescence

66. _____ senescence

67. _____ progeria

68. _____ gerontology

CHAPTER 34

Genetics and Heredity

Look about your classroom and you will notice various combinations of hair color, eye color, body size, skin tone, hair texture, sex, etc. Everyone has unique body features and this phenomenon alerts us to the marvel of genetics. Independent units, called *genes*, are responsible for the inheritance of biological traits. Genes determine the structure and function of the human body by producing specific regulatory enzymes. Some genes are dominant and some are recessive. Dominant genes produce traits that appear in the offspring and recessive genes have traits that do not appear in the offspring when they are masked by a dominant gene.

Gene therapy is one of the latest advances of science. This revolutionary branch of medicine combines current technology with genetic research to unlock the secrets of the human body. Daily discoveries into the prevention, diagnosis, treatment, and cure of diseases and disorders are being revealed as a result of genetic therapy. A knowledge of genetics is necessary to understand the basic mechanism by which traits are transmitted from parents to offspring.

I—THE SCIENCE OF GENETICS; CHROMOSOMES AND GENES; GENE EXPRESSION

Multiple Choice—select the best answer.

1. When its genetic codes are being expressed, DNA is in a threadlike form called:
   a. mRNA.
   b. chromosomes.
   c. chromatin.
   d. tRNA.

2. DNA is arranged to form a larger structure called a:
   a. gene.
   b. genome.
   c. chromosome.
   d. gamete.

3. A person with a genotype expressed as *AA* is said to be:
   a. heterozygous recessive.
   b. heterozygous dominant.
   c. homozygous recessive.
   d. homozygous dominant.

4. Both males and females need at least:
   a. one normal Y chromosome.
   b. two normal X chromosomes.
   c. one normal X chromosome.
   d. two normal Y chromosomes.

5. The entire collection of genetic material in each typical cell of the human body is called the:
   a. genome.
   b. chromosome.
   c. genotype.
   d. phenotype.

6. Mutations are caused:
   a. spontaneously.
   b. by mutagens.
   c. by environmental agents that damage DNA.
   d. all of the above.

7. Red-green color blindness is an example of an X-linked recessive condition. If X is normal, X1 is recessive, and Y is normal, an individual with the genotype XX1 will be:
   a. a normal male.
   b. a color-blind male.
   c. a normal female and a carrier.
   d. a normal female and not a carrier.

8. The scientific study of genetics began in the:
   a. 16th century.
   b. 17th century.
   c. 18th century.
   d. 19th century.

True or false

9. ___F___ Each of the 23 pairs of chromosomes always appear to be nearly identical to each other.

10. ___T___ The manner in which genotype is expressed is termed *phenotype*.

11. ___F___ *Sickle-cell trait* and *sickle-cell anemia* are synonymous terms.

12. ___F___ Normal males have the sex chromosome combination XX, whereas normal females have the sex chromosome combination XY.

13. ___T___ X-linked recessive traits appear much more frequently in males than in females.

14. _____ Statistical evidence supports the notion that having sexual intercourse on the day of ovulation increases the probability of conceiving a male.

15. _____ Each cell of the body, except gametes, contains 46 pairs of chromosomes.

16. _____ A person whose genotype is heterozygous for albinism will express the abnormal phenotype of albinism.

▷ *If you had difficulty with this section, review pages 1200-1209.*

II—MEDICAL GENETICS; PREVENTION AND TREATMENT OF GENETIC DISEASES

Multiple Choice—select the best answer.

17. Trisomy and monosomy result from:
    a. an error in meiosis called *disjunction.*
    b. an error in meiosis called *nondisjunction.*
    c. single-gene abnormality.
    d. chromosome breakage.

18. Trisomy 21 is also called:
    a. Klinefelter syndrome.
    b. Down syndrome.
    c. Turner syndrome.
    d. cystic fibrosis.

19. A person with the sex chromosomes XXY is afflicted with:
    a. Klinefelter syndrome.
    b. Down syndrome.
    c. Turner syndrome.
    d. cystic fibrosis.

20. Which of the following is *NOT* a recessive X-linked genetic disease?
    a. hemophilia
    b. red-green color blindness
    c. sickle-cell anemia
    d. cleft palate

21. Which of the following abnormal genes are linked to some form of cancer?
    a. codominant genes
    b. tumor suppressor genes
    c. oncogenes
    d. recessive genes

22. A grid used to determine the mathematical probability of inheriting genetic traits is called:
    a. a pedigree.
    b. a Punnett square.
    c. amniocentesis.
    d. a chorionic villus sampling.

23. Which of the following genetic diseases can be treated to some degree, if diagnosed early?
    a. PKU
    b. Turner syndrome
    c. Klinefelter syndrome
    d. all of the above

24. In gene replacement therapy:
    a. genetically altered cells are introduced into the body.
    b. genetic disease is treated by inducing an alteration in metabolism.
    c. synthetic hormones are used to relieve symptoms.
    d. genes that specify production of abnormal, disease-causing proteins are replaced by normal or "therapeutic" genes.

25. Disorders that involve trisomy or monosomy can be detected after a _____ is produced.
    a. genotype
    b. phenotype
    c. karyotype
    d. polytype

26. Cells that display distinct chromosomes during collection via amniocentesis and chorionic villus sampling are in:
    a. prophase.
    b. metaphase.
    c. anaphase.
    d. telophase.

True or false

27. _____ *Congenital disorders* and *inherited disorders* are synonymous terms.

28. _____ Sickle-cell trait is milder than sickle-cell anemia.

29. _____ Parkinson disease is linked to an error in the nuclear DNA.

30. _____ A pedigree is a chart that illustrates genetic relationships in a family over several generations.

31. _____ Electrophoresis is a method for determining an individual's DNA sequence, or DNA "fingerprint."

32. _____ Cystic fibrosis is a blood-clotting disorder.

33. _____ Cleft palate is a recessive X-linked disorder.

34. _____ Chorionic villus sampling is a procedure newer than amniocentesis.

35. _____ "Genes are not there to cause disease."

▷ *If you had difficulty with this section, review pages 1209-1223.*

Crossword Puzzle

Across

2. Having half of the normal chromosomes
8. Triplet of autosomes
9. Entire collection of genetic material in each cell
10. Grid used to predict genetic traits (two words)

Down

1. Used to identify chromosomal disorders
3. Having a characteristic pair of chromosomes
4. Presence of one autosome
5. Equal effect of different dominant genes
6. Genotype with two identical forms of a gene
7. One of the 44 chromosomes (excluding sex chromosomes)

APPLYING WHAT YOU KNOW

36. Deb's mother has a dominant gene for dark skin color. Her father has a dominant gene for light skin color. What color will Deb's skin most likely be?

37. Mr. and Mrs. Mihm both carry recessive genes for cystic fibrosis. Using your knowledge of the Punnett square, estimate the probability of one of their offspring inheriting this condition.

DID YOU KNOW?

* Scientists estimate that they could fill a 1000-volume encyclopedia with the coded instructions in the DNA of a single human cell if the instructions could be translated into English.

* Identical twins do not have identical fingerprints. No two sets of prints are alike, including those of identical twins.

ONE LAST QUICK CHECK

Multiple Choice—select the best answer.

38. Independent assortment of chromosomes ensures:
    a. each offspring from a single set of parents is genetically unique.
    b. at meiosis each gamete receives the same number of chromosomes.
    c. that the sex chromosomes always match.
    d. an equal number of males and females are born.

39. Which of the following statements is *NOT* true of a pedigree?
    a. They are useful to genetic counselors in predicting the possibility of producing offspring with genetic disorders.
    b. They may allow a person to determine his or her likelihood of developing a genetic disorder later in life.
    c. They indicate the occurrence of those family members affected by a trait, as well as carriers of the trait.
    d. All of the above are true of a pedigree.

40. The genes that cause albinism are:
    a. codominant.
    b. dominant.
    c. recessive.
    d. AA.

41. During meiosis, matching pairs of chromosomes line up and exchange genes from their location to the same location on the other side; a process called:
    a. gene linkage.
    b. crossing-over.
    c. cross-linkage.
    d. genetic variation.

42. When a sperm cell unites with an ovum, a _____ is formed.
    a. zygote
    b. chromosome
    c. gamete
    d. none of the above

43. DNA molecules can also be called:
    a. a chromatin strand.
    b. a chromosome.
    c. a and b.
    d. none of the above.

44. Sex-linked traits:
    a. show up more often in females than in males.
    b. are nonsexual traits carried on sex chromosomes.
    c. are the result of genetic mutation.
    d. all of the above.

45. If a person has only X chromosomes, that person is:
    a. missing essential proteins.
    b. abnormal.
    c. female.
    d. male.

46. A karyotype:
    a. can detect trisomy.
    b. is useful for diagnosing a tubal pregnancy.
    c. is frequently used as a tool in gene augmentation therapy.
    d. can detect the presence of oncogenes.

47. Which of the following pairs is mismatched?
    a. osteogenesis imperfecta—dominant
    b. Turner syndrome—trisomy
    c. PKU—recessive
    d. cystic fibrosis—recessive

Completion—using the terms below, complete the following statements.

a. cystic fibrosis
b. males
c. phenylketonuria
d. carrier
e. genome
f. females
g. dominant
h. oncogenes
i. karyotype
j. Tay-Sachs disease
k. amniocentesis
l. hemophilia

48. Abnormal genes called _____ are believed to be related to cancer.

49. Fetal tissue may be collected by a procedure called _____.

50. An abnormal accumulation of phenylalanine results in _____.

51. The entire collection of genetic material in each cell is called the _____.

52. _____ is caused by recessive genes in chromosome pair seven.

53. A _____ is a person who has a recessive gene that is not expressed.

54. Absence of an essential lipid-producing enzyme may result in the recessive condition _____.

55. _____ is a recessive X-linked disorder characterized as a blood clotting disorder.

56. A gene capable of masking the effects of a recessive gene for the same trait is a _____ gene.

Answer Key

CHAPTER 1

Anatomy and Physiology and Characteristics of Life
1. b, p. 7
2. c, p. 7
3. a, p. 7
4. b, p. 8
5. c, p. 9

Levels of Organization
6. d, p. 10
7. a, p. 9
8. c, p. 9
9. c, p. 11
10. c, p. 12
11. d, p. 9
12. e, p. 9
13. a, p. 9
14. c, p. 11
15. b, p. 11
16. a, p. 11
17. a, p. 11
18. a, p. 11
19. b, p. 11
20. b, p. 11
21. e, p. 11
22. e, p. 11
23. d, p. 11
24. d, p. 11
25. e, p. 11
26. c, p. 11

Anatomical Position, Body Cavities, Body Regions, Anatomical Terms, and Body Planes
27. b, p. 12
28. a, p. 13
29. a, p. 13
30. d, p. 15
31. c, p. 13
32. c, p. 13
33. b, p. 14
34. b, p. 18

35. c, p. 18
36. d, p. 15
37. inferior, p. 17
38. anterior, p. 17
39. lateral, p. 17
40. proximal, p. 17
41. superficial, p. 17
42. equal, p. 18
43. anterior and posterior, p. 18
44. upper and lower, p. 18
45. frontal, p. 18
46. a, p. 13
47. b, p. 13
48. a, p. 13
49. a, p. 13
50. a, p. 13
51. a, p. 13

Homeostasis and Homeostatic Mechanisms of Control
52. a, p. 22
53. d, p. 24
54. a, p. 25
55. b, p. 26
56. f, p. 24
57. f, p. 24
58. t, p. 25
59. t, p. 27

Health Matters
60. b, p. 29
61. e, p. 29
62. a, p. 29
63. d, p. 29
64. c, p. 29
65. f, p. 29
66. h, p. 29
67. i, p. 29
68. g, p. 29
69. j, p. 29
70. pathophysiology
71. homeostasis
72. mutated

73. parasite
74. tumors
75. self-immunity

Applying What You Know
76. #1 on diagram
77. #2 on diagram
78. #3 on diagram

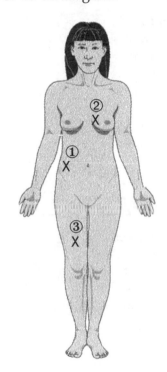

One Last Quick Check
79. a, p. 22
80. d, p. 16
81. d, p. 18
82. a, p. 7
83. b, p. 16
84. d, p. 13
85. d, p. 17
86. d, p. 15
87. a, p. 15
88. c, p. 17

Diagrams

Directions and Planes of the Body

1. transverse plane
2. lateral plane
3. coronal plane
4. medial
5. sagittal plane
6. inferior
7. distal
8. proximal
9. anterior (ventral)
10. superior
11. posterior (dorsal)

Body Cavities

1. cranial
2. spinal
3. pleural
4. thoracic
5. abdominal
6. pelvic
7. ventral
8. dorsal

CHAPTER 2

Basic Chemistry

1. c, p. 38
2. c, p. 38
3. c, p. 38
4. d, p. 40
5. c, p. 41
6. c, p. 43
7. b, p. 44
8. a, p. 45
9. t, p. 38
10. t, p. 39
11. f, p. 43
12. f, p. 44
13. t, p. 45
14. oxygen
15. calcium
16. potassium
17. sodium
18. magnesium
19. iron
20. selenium

Metabolism

21. a, p. 46
22. d, p. 46
23. b, p. 46
24. c, p. 45
25. e, p. 46

Inorganic Molecules

26. d, p. 47
27. d, p. 47
28. c, p. 49
29. b, p. 49
30. c, p. 49
31. t, p. 49
32. t, p. 50
33. t, p. 49
34. t, p. 46
35. f, p. 47

Organic Molecules

36. c, p. 53
37. d, p. 51
38. c, p. 54
39. a, p. 54
40. c, p. 57
41. b, p. 63
42. c, p. 67
43. d, p. 66
44. a, p. 66
45. f, p. 63
46. t, p. 65
47. f, p. 57
48. t, p. 54
49. t, p. 53
50. t, p. 65

Applying What You Know

51. (A) Basement (B) Increasing ventilation or sealing the basement floors
52. Unsaturated fats can often form a solid mass at higher temperatures. Review pages 62 and 63 for more information.

One Last Quick Check

53. e, p. 41
54. b, p. 67
55. g, p. 41
56. a, p. 38
57. i, p. 53
58. f, p. 66
59. h, p. 47
60. c, p. 48
61. b, p. 53
62. c, p. 63
63. a, p. 54
64. c, p. 63
65. b, p. 53
66. c, p. 63
67. a, p. 53
68. b, p. 49
69. a, p. 49
70. b, p. 49
71. b, p. 49
72. a, p. 49

CHAPTER 3

Functional Anatomy of Cells

1. b, p. 82
2. d, p. 84
3. b, p. 89
4. d, p. 92
5. a, p. 89
6. a, p. 92
7. b, p. 93
8. f, p. 84
9. f, p. 93
10. f, p. 92
11. t, p. 92
12. f, p. 80
13. a, p. 93
14. d, p. 82
15. b, p. 91
16. f, p. 89
17. c, p. 82
18. h, p. 92
19. g, p. 92
20. e, p. 96

Cytoskeleton

21. cytoskeleton, p. 93
22. microfilaments, p. 94
23. microtubules, p. 94
24. centrosome, p. 94
25. microvilli, cilia, flagella, p. 95
26. gap junctions, p. 97
27. desmosomes, p. 97

Applying What You Know

28. (a) CD 36 (b) LDL (c) stroke, diabetes, cancer, muscular dystrophy
29. mitochondria

One Last Quick Check
30. b, p. 95
31. c, p. 96
32. b, p. 97
33. b, p. 88
34. b, p. 84
35. e, p. 81
36. d, p. 81
37. b, p. 81
38. a, p. 81
39. c, p. 81
40. composite, p. 82
41. hydrophilic, p. 84
42. signal transduction, p. 86
43. peroxisomes, p. 91
44. nucleus, p. 92

Diagrams

Microscope
1. ocular lens
2. mechanical stage
3. condenser lens
4. coarse focus
5. fine focus
6. light source
7. specimen on slide
8. objective lens

Cell Anatomy
1. centrosome
2. smooth endoplasmic reticulum
3. rough endoplasmic reticulum
4. nuclear envelope
5. nucleolus
6. microvilli
7. Golgi apparatus
8. cilia
9. mitochondria
10. ribosomes

CHAPTER 4

Movement of Substances Through Cell Membranes
1. d, p. 112
2. b, p. 105
3. c, p. 105
4. a, p. 108
5. b, p. 110
6. f, p. 109
7. t, p. 111
8. t, p. 114
9. t, p. 107
10. f, p. 106
11. b, p. 108
12. a, p. 108
13. c, p. 108
14. d, p. 104
15. e, p. 111

Cell Metabolism
16. b, p. 114
17. a, p. 122
18. c, p. 123
19. b, p. 124
20. c, p. 121
21. d, p. 123
22. t, p. 117
23. t, p. 114
24. f, p. 123
25. f, p. 122
26. t, p. 120
27. t, p. 118
28. f, p. 118
29. e, p. 123
30. a, p. 125
31. c, p. 125
32. d, p. 125
33. f, p. 123
34. b, p. 125

Growth and Reproduction of Cells
35. a, p. 130
36. a, p. 130
37. b, p. 133
38. c, p. 136
39. f, p. 132
40. t, p. 130
41. f, p. 133
42. t, p. 131
43. f, p. 136

Mechanisms of Disease
44. t, p. 138
45. t, p. 138
46. t, p. 138
47. f, p. 139
48. t, p. 138

Applying What You Know
49. diffusion
50. shrink

One Last Quick Check
51. b, p. 131
52. a, p. 125
53. a, p. 111
54. d, p. 104
55. d, p. 106
56. a, p. 115
57. c, p. 117
58. b, p. 110
59. c, p. 110
60. c, p. 111
61. a, p. 105
62. b, p. 108
63. a, p. 108
64. uracil (RNA contains the base uracil, not DNA)
65. thymine (the others refer to RNA)
66. interphase (the others refer to translation)
67. prophase (the others refer to anaphase)
68. gene (the others refer to stages of cell division)

Diagrams

Cellular Respiration
1. glucose
2. acetyl-CoA
3. citric acid cycle
4. mitochondrion
5. ATP
6. oxygen O_2
7. water H_2O
8. aerobic
9. anaerobic
10. transition
11. pyruvic acid
12. lactic acid

DNA Molecule
1. hydrogen bonds
2. sugar
3. phosphate
4. cytosine
5. guanine
6. adenine
7. thymine

Mitosis
1. prophase
2. metaphase
3. anaphase
4. telophase

CHAPTER 5

Principal Types of Tissues
1. b, p. 146
2. c, p. 146
3. d, p. 146
4. b, p. 146
5. b, p. 146
6. a, p. 146
7. t, p. 146
8. t, p. 146
9. f, p. 147
10. t, p. 146

Epithelial Tissue
11. d, p. 150
12. b, p. 151
13. b, p. 151
14. b, p. 150
15. c, p. 152
16. b, p. 157
17. a, p. 159
18. d, p. 159
19. a, p. 151
20. t, p. 150
21. f, p. 150
22. f, p. 157
23. b, p. 151
24. e, p. 152
25. d, p. 152
26. h, p. 155
27. a, p. 151
28. c, p. 152

Connective Tissue
29. a, p. 161
30. c, p. 160
31. b, p. 161
32. d, p. 162
33. c, p. 164
34. d, p. 170
35. a, p. 170
36. b, p. 170
37. a, p. 172
38. d, p. 167

39. t, p. 161
40. t, p. 170
41. f, p. 170
42. f, p. 170
43. t, p. 160
44. f, p. 166

Muscle Tissue
45. b, p. 175
46. c, p. 177
47. a, p. 177
48. b, p. 175
49. c, p. 175
50. c, p. 175

Nervous Tissue
51. d, p. 177
52. b, p. 177
53. c, p. 177
54. a, p. 177
55. e, p. 177

Tissue Repair
56. h, p. 167
57. d, p. 167
58. b, p. 178
59. a, p. 167
60. j, p. 167
61. f, p. 167
62. e, p. 167
63. g, p. 178
64. i, p. 167
65. c, p. 167

Body Membranes
66. a, p. 179
67. b, p. 181
68. f, p. 179
69. t, p. 181

Tumors and Cancer
70. slowly, p. 183
71. are not, p. 183
72. papilloma, p. 183
73. sarcoma, p. 184
74. oncologist, p. 184
75. cytotoxic, p. 185

Applying What You Know
76. Too lean. Holly should be in the 20–22% range to be considered normal. Hol-ly's obsession may put her at risk for other disease conditions because of the stress to her body of being "too lean."
77. Modalities—medical imaging, biopsy, and blood tests
Tissues—epithelial, connective, and muscle

One Last Quick Check
78. squamous, p. 151
79. cuboidal, p. 151
80. columnar, p. 151
81. simple squamous, p. 151
82. simple cuboidal, p. 151
83. simple columnar, p. 151
84. stratified (transitional), p. 151
85. pseudostratified, p. 151
86. a, p. 146
87. d, p. 155
88. b, p. 160
89. c, p. 161
90. c, p. 164
91. b, p. 172
92. a, p. 179
93. c, p. 179

Diagrams

Tissue #1 is epithelial
1. basement membrane
2. cell nuclei
3. cuboidal epithelial cells
4. lumen of tubule

Tissue #2 is simple columnar epithelial
1. goblet cells
2. columnar epithelial cell

Tissue #3 is pseudostratified ciliated epithelium
1. cilia
2. columnar cell
3. goblet cell
4. basement membrane
5. mucous glands

Tissue#4 is stratified squamous (keratinized) epithelium
1. cornified layer
2. basement membrane
3. basal cells
4. dermis

Tissue #5 is loose, ordinary (areolar) connective
1. bundle of collagenous fibers
2. elastic fibers

Tissue #6 is adipose
1. storage area for fat
2. plasma membrane
3. nucleus of adipose

Tissue #7 is dense fibrous (regular) connective
1. fibroblast
2. collagenous fibers

Tissue #8 is elastic cartilage
1. lacuna
2. chondrocyte
3. elastic fibers

Tissue # 9 is bone
1. osteon (Haversian system)

Tissue # 10 is skeletal muscle
1. cross striations of muscle cell
2. nuclei of muscle cell
3. muscle fiber

Tissue # 11 is cardiac muscle
1. nucleus
2. intercalated disks

Tissue # 12 is nervous
1. nerve cell body
2. axon
3. dendrites

CHAPTER 6

Skin Function and Structure
1. b, p. 196
2. a, p. 197
3. d, p. 198
4. d, p. 199
5. a, p. 198
6. d, p. 202
7. c, p. 217
8. c, p. 203
9. b, p. 204
10. c, p. 204
11. f, p. 196
12. t, p. 203
13. t, p. 204
14. f, p. 217
15. t, p. 201

Functions of the Skin
16. d, p. 208
17. d, p. 208
18. c, p. 209
19. a, p. 209
20. b, p. 210
21. f, p. 209
22. f, p. 208
23. t, p. 210

Appendages of the Skin
24. b, p. 210
25. a, p. 213
26. c, p. 215
27. b, p. 214
28. d, p. 213
29. t, p. 211
30. f, p. 212
31. t, p. 214
32. t, p. 213
33. t, p. 214

Skin Disorders
34. f, p. 216
35. c, p. 216
36. a, p. 218
37. b, p. 218
38. g, p. 219
39. h, p. 220
40. d, p. 220
41. e, p. 220
42. Fever or febrile, p. 221
43. Heat exhaustion, p. 222
44. Heat stroke, p. 221
45. Frostbite c, p. 222

Burns
46. a, p. 222
47. b, p. 223
48. f, p. 222
49. t, p. 222
50. c, p. 222
51. a, p. 221
52. d, p. 221
53. b, p. 221
54. e, p. 221

Applying What You Know
55. 46%
56. fingerprints
57. It is theorized that adults who had more than two blistering sunburns before the age of 20 have a greater risk of developing melanoma than someone who experienced no burns.
Bernie's exposure may have been during his youth or adolescence.

One Last Quick Check
58. a, p. 202
59. d, p. 215
60. b, p. 204
61. d, p. 222
62. b, p. 215
63. b, p. 197
64. c, p. 213
65. b, p. 207
66. a, p. 201
67. a, p. 199
68. c, p. 204
69. b, p. 203
70. e, p. 215
71. f, p. 210
72. g, p. 213
73. a, p. 201
74. d, p. 214
75. h, p. 215
76. i, p. 216
77. j, p. 220

Diagrams

Skin
1. opening of sweat ducts
2. hair shaft
3. stratum corneum
4. stratum granulosum
5. stratum basale

6. dermal papilla
7. Meissner's corpuscle
8. sebaceous (oil) gland
9. hair follicle
10. hypodermis
11. dermis
12. epidermis

Rule of Nines
1. 4.5%
2. 4.5%
3. 18%
4. 4.5%
5. 1%
6. 9%
7. 9%
8. 9%
9. 9%
10. 4.5%
11. 4.5%
12. 18%
13. 4.5%

CHAPTER 7

Types of Bones
1. f, p. 232
2. k, p. 230
3. h, p. 231
4. e, p. 230
5. d, p. 231
6. i, p. 230
7. j, p. 231
8. c, p. 230
9. a, p. 231
10. b, p. 231
11. g, p. 231

Bone Tissue Structure, Function, and Homeostasis
12. d, p. 232
13. b, p. 233
14. c, p. 233
15. b, p. 236
16. b, p. 237
17. c, p. 237
18. t, p. 235
19. f, p. 236
20. t, p. 237
21. t, p. 238
22. f, p. 237

23. f, p. 237

Bone Development, Growth, Resorption, and Repair
24. b, p. 240
25. d, p. 240
26. a, p. 240
27. b, p. 242
28. b, p. 243
29. t, p. 238
30. f, p. 238
31. f, p. 242
32. t, p. 238
33. t, p. 241

Cartilage
34. b, p. 244
35. c, p. 245
36. b, p. 248
37. f, p. 244
38. t, p. 245
39. t, p. 246

Mechanisms of Disease
40. Chondrosarcoma
41. Osteosarcoma
42. Osteoporosis
43. Paget's disease
44. Osteomyelitis

Applying What You Know
45. (a) Osteoporosis
  (b) DXA—dual energy x-ray absorptiometry scan or bone density (RA) imagery of the wrist
  (c) hormonal therapy (HRT), bone-building nonhormonal drugs such as Fosamax or Miacalcin, vitamin (D) and mineral (calcium) therapy, and weight-bearing exercises.
46. The bones are responsible for the majority of our blood cell formation. Her disease condition might be inhibiting the production of blood cells.
47. Epiphyseal cartilage is present only while a child is still growing. It be-

comes bone in adulthood. It is particularly vulnerable to fractures in childhood and preadolescence.
48. Ms. Strickland's surgeon most likely used a synthetic skeletal repair material called "vitos" which facilitates fracture repairs. Unlike metal stabilizers, vitos "patches" degrade naturally in the body following surgery and do not require surgical removal.

One Last Quick Check
49. four, p. 230
50. medullary cavity, p. 231
51. articular cartilage, p. 231
52. endosteum, p. 232
53. hematopoiesis, p. 237
54. red bone marrow, p. 237
55. periosteum, p. 231
56. long, short, flat, and irregular, p. 230
57. calcium, p. 237
58. hyaline, p. 245
59. d, p. 235
60. b, p. 230
61. e, p. 231
62. a, p. 231
63. c, p. 244
64. i, p. 236
65. f, p. 233
66. j, p. 233
67. g, p. 244
68. h, p. 233

Diagrams

Long Bone
1. epiphysis
2. diaphysis
3. epiphysis
4. periosteum
5. yellow marrow
6. endosteum
7. medullary cavity
8. compact bone
9. red marrow cavities
10. epiphyseal plate

11. spongy bone
12. articular cartilage

Cross-Section of Cancellous and Compact Bone
1. osteons (Haversian systems)
2. periosteum
3. compact bone
4. medullary marrow cavity
5. Volkmann's canals
6. Haversian canals
7. trabeculae
8. endosteum

CHAPTER 8

Divisions of the Skeleton
1. a, p. 257
2. a, p. 257
3. b, p. 256
4. a, p. 257
5. b, p. 257
6. b, p. 257
7. a, p. 257
8. b, p. 257
9. a, p. 257
10. b, p. 257

The Skull
11. c, p. 256
12. d, p. 256
13. a, p. 256
14. c, p. 257
15. a, p. 274
16. b, p. 265
17. f, p. 257
18. f, p. 276
19. t, p. 274
20. f, p. 276
21. t, p. 272

Sternum and Ribs
22. e, p. 285
23. c, p. 285
24. a, p. 284
25. d, p. 284
26. f, p. 284
27. b, p. 285
28. g, p. 284

The Appendicular Skeleton/

Upper Extremity
29. b, p. 286
30. d, p. 287
31. d, p. 287
32. t, p. 286
33. f, p. 289
34. t, p. 288
35. f, p. 289

The Appendicular Skeleton/ Lower Extremity
36. b, p. 292
37. a, p. 293
38. a, p. 292
39. c, p. 293
40. f, p. 292
41. f, p. 290
42. f, p. 290
43. f, p. 295

Skeletal Differences in Men and Women
44. b, p. 297
45. a, p. 297
46. a, p. 297
47. b, p. 297
48. a, p. 297
49. b, p. 297

Cycle of Life: Mechanisms of Disease
50. b, p. 300
51. c, p. 299
52. f, p. 303
53. t, p. 303

Applying What You Know
54. Bill could have possibly injured his humerus and his ulna.
55. (a) High heels cause a forward thrust to the body which forces an undue amount of weight on the heads of the metatarsals. (b) Metatarsals, tarsals, and phalanges

One Last Quick Check
56. coxal (all others refer to the spine)
57. axial (all others refer to the appendicular skeleton)
58. maxilla (all others refer to the cranial bones)
59. ribs (all others refer to the shoulder girdle)
60. vomer (all others refer to the bones of the middle ear)
61. ulna (all others refer to the coxal bone)
62. ethmoid (all others refer to the hand and wrist)
63. nasal (all others refer to cranial bones)
64. anvil (all others refer to the cervical vertebra)
65. c, p. 273
66. g, p. 279
67. j, l, m, k, p. 289
68. n, p. 290
69. i, p. 279 and 287
70. a, p. 272
71. p, p. 290
72. b, d, p. 272
73. f, p. 273
74. h, q, p. 287
75. o, t, p. 290
76. r, p. 272
77. s, e, p. 273

Diagrams

Anterior View of Skull
1. glabella
2. ethmoid bone
3. sphenoid bone
4. nasal bone
5. vomer
6. mental foramen
7. mandible
8. maxilla
9. perpendicular plate of ethmoid
10. optic foramen
11. parietal bone
12. frontal bone

Floor of Cranial Cavity
1. crista galli
2. optic foramen
3. internal auditory meatus
4. jugular foramen

5. foramen magnum
6. occipital bone
7. petrous portion of temporal bone
8. sella turcica
9. greater wing of sphenoid bone
10. lesser wing of sphenoid bone

Skull Viewed from Below
1. palatine process of maxilla
2. zygomatic arch
3. foramen ovale
4. styloid process
5. occipital condyle
6. foramen magnum
7. horizontal plate of palatine
8. zygomatic process of maxilla
9. hard palate
10. incisive foramen

Left Half of Skull
1. squamous suture
2. parietal bone
3. lambdoidal suture
4. temporal bone (squamous portion)
5. occipital bone
6. external auditory meatus
7. condyloid process
8. mastoid process of temporal bone
9. styloid process
10. pterygoid process
11. coronoid process
12. mandible
13. mental foramen
14. maxilla
15. zygomatic (malar) bone
16. nasal bone
17. lacrimal bone
18. ethmoid bone
19. sphenoid bone
20. frontal bone
21. coronal suture

Bones that Form the Orbit
1. optic foramen
2. superior orbital fissure

3. ethmoid bone
4. lacrimal bone
5. maxilla
6. inferior orbital fissure
7. infraorbital foramen
8. zygomatic bone
9. sphenoid bone
10. frontal bone

Skull at Birth
1. parietal bone
2. occipital fontanel
3. occipital bone
4. mastoid fontanel
5. sphenoid fontanel
6. sagittal suture
7. occipital fontanel
8. occipital bone
9. parietal bone
10. coronal suture
11. frontal fontanel
12. frontal bone
13. coronal suture
14. frontal fontanel

The Vertebral Column
1. thoracic curvature
2. intervertebral foramina
3. pelvic curvature
4. atlas
5. axis
6. cervical curvature
7. lumbar curvature
8. coccyx
9. sacrum
10. lumbar vertebrae
11. thoracic vertebrae
12. cervical vertebrae

Vertebrae Atlas
1. transverse process
2. transverse foramen
3. anterior arch
4. facet for dens
5. vertebral foramen
6. superior articular facet
7. posterior arch

Cervical Vertebra
1. spinous process
2. lamina
3. pedicle
4. transverse foramen
5. transverse process

6. superior articular facet
7. vertebral foramen

Lumbar Vertebra
1. spinous process
2. lamina
3. transverse process
4. pedicle
5. superior articular facet
6. vertebral foramen

Axis
1. spinous process
2. transverse process
3. transverse foramen
4. dens
5. superior articular facet
6. vertebral foramen
7. posterior arch

Thoracic Vertebra
1. spinous process
2. lamina
3. transverse process
4. pedicle
5. superior articular facet
6. articular facet for tubercle of rib
7. vertebral foramen

Sacrum and Coccyx
1. superior articular facet
2. articular surface
3. median sacral crest
4. sacral foramina
5. sacral hiatus
6. coccyx
7. sacrum
8. ala
9. sacral canal

Thoracic Cage
1. clavicle
2. true ribs
3. costal cartilage
4. costosternal articulation
5. false ribs
6. floating ribs
7. xiphoid process
8. body
9. manubrium
10. sternum
11. first thoracic vertebra
12. seventh cervical vertebra

Rib

1. rib
2. head
3. neck
4. transverse process
5. sternal extremity
6. body
7. angle
8. nonarticular part of tubercle
9. neck
10. head
11. vertebral extremity
12. articular part of tubercle

Scapula Anterior View

1. superior angle
2. superior border
3. coracoid process
4. acromion process
5. supraglenoid tubercle
6. glenoid cavity
7. infraglenoid tubercle
8. axillary border
9. inferior angle
10. vertebral border
11. costal surface

Posterior View

1. acromion process
2. coracoid process
3. spine
4. superior border
5. medial angle
6. vertebral border
7. inferior angle
8. dorsal surface
9. axillary border
10. glenoid cavity

Lateral View

1. coracoid process
2. glenoid cavity
3. infraglenoid tubercle
4. axillary border
5. inferior angle

Bones of the Arm Anterior View

1. humerus
2. greater tubercle
3. lesser tubercle
4. lateral epicondyle
5. capitulum
6. coronoid fossa
7. medial epicondyle
8. styloid process of radius
9. radial tuberosity
10. radius
11. olecranon process
12. styloid process of ulna

Posterior View

1. head
2. anatomical neck
3. trochlea
4. olecranon fossa
5. coronoid process
6. head of radius
7. olecranon process

Bones of the Hand and Wrist

1. carpal bones
2. ulna
3. phalanges
4. metacarpal
5. radius

Coxal Bone

1. ilium
2. greater sciatic notch
3. ischium
4. obturator foramen
5. ischial tuberosity
6. pubis
7. acetabulum
8. iliac crest

Bones of the Thigh and Leg

1. greater trochanter
2. lateral epicondyle
3. medial epicondyle
4. femur
5. lesser trochanter
6. intertrochanteric line
7. neck
8. head
9. medial condyle
10. head of fibula
11. fibula
12. lateral malleolus
13. medial malleolus
14. tibia
15. crest
16. tibial tuberosity
17. medial condyle
18. intercondylar eminence

Foot

1. phalanges
2. metatarsals
3. tarsals
4. navicular
5. talus
6. calcaneus
7. cuboid

CHAPTER 9

Classification of Joints

1. b, p. 312
2. a, p. 314
3. a, p. 312
4. c, p. 314
5. c, p. 313
6. d, p. 314
7. c, p. 316
8. d, p. 316
9. t, p. 314
10. f, p. 314
11. t, p. 316
12. t, p. 312
13. f, p. 314
14. f, p. 312
15. f, p. 314
16. t, p. 316
17. a, p. 313
18. a, p. 312
19. b, p. 316
20. c, p. 312
21. c, p. 312
22. a, p. 312
23. b, p. 316
24. c, p. 312
25. b, p. 312
26. b, p. 314
27. a, p. 312
28. b, p. 314
29. d, p. 316
30. c, p. 316
31. b, p. 316
32. e, p. 316
33. d, p. 316
34. c, p. 316
35. a, p. 316

36. a, p. 316
37. f, p. 316

Representative Synovial Joints
38. c, p. 317
39. b, p. 324
40. b, p. 324
41. a, p. 324
42. d, p. 327
43. c, p. 327
44. b, p. 324
45. c, p. 338

Types and Range of Movement at Synovial Joints
46. e, p. 330
47. c, p. 336
48. f, p. 336
49. g, p. 330
50. b, p. 330
51. d, p. 330
52. a, p. 336
53. h, p. 336
54. i, p. 336
55. j, p. 336

Mechanisms of Disease
56. arthroscopy
57. osteoarthritis or degenerative joint disease
58. arthritis
59. gouty arthritis
60. sprain

Applying What You Know
61. (a) Nodular swelling, joint pain, tenderness, aching, stiffness, and limited motion. Systemic symptoms may also include fever, anemia, weight loss, profound fatigue, and possible pericarditis.
(b) Small joints of the hand, wrist, and feet progressing often to the larger joints.
62. (a) Gouty arthritis
(b) Swelling, tenderness, and pain, typically in the joints of the fingers, wrists, elbows, ankles, and knees.
(c) Allopurinol (Zyloprim) is the drug of choice to treat this disease.

One Last Quick Check
63. diarthroses
64. synarthrotic
65. diarthrotic
66. ligaments
67. articular cartilage
68. least movable
69. largest
70. 2
71. mobility
72. pivot
73. t, p. 314
74. f, p. 312
75. f, p. 337
76. t, p. 319
77. t, p. 330
78. t, p. 336
79. f, p. 336
80. f, p. 336
81. f, p. 341
82. t, p. 324

Diagrams

Synovial Joint
1. bursa
2. articular cartilage
3. periosteum
4. joint capsule
5. nerve
6. synovial membrane
7. bone
8. joint cavity

Shoulder Joint
1. coracoid process of scapula
2. glenoid cavity
3. superior transverse ligament of scapula
4. articular cartilage of glenoid cavity
5. scapula
6. glenoidal labrum
7. humerus
8. head of humerus
9. articular cartilage of humerus
10. bursa
11. tendon of long head of biceps brachii m.
12. synovial cavity

Hip Joint
1. acetabular labrum
2. head
3. articular capsule
4. greater trochanter
5. femur
6. lesser trochanter
7. articular capsule
8. transverse acetabular ligament
9. ligamentum teres
10. articular cavity
11. acetabulum
12. ilium

Knee Joint Anterior View
1. lateral condyle of femur
2. lateral meniscus
3. fibular collateral ligament
4. transverse ligament of knee
5. fibula
6. tibia
7. tibial tuberosity
8. tibial collateral ligament
9. medial meniscus
10. anterior cruciate ligament
11. medial condyle of femur
12. posterior cruciate ligament
13. femur

Knee Joint Posterior View
1. femur
2. ligament of Wrisberg
3. medial condyle
4. medial meniscus
5. tibial collateral ligament
6. posterior cruciate ligament
7. tibia
8. fibula
9. fibular collateral ligament
10. lateral meniscus
11. lateral condyle

12. anterior cruciate ligament

Vertebrae
1. lamina
2. anterior longitudinal ligament
3. body of vertebra
4. intervertebral disk
5. posterior longitudinal ligament
6. ligamentum flavum
7. intervertebral foramen

CHAPTER 10

Skeletal Muscle Structure
1. c, p. 348
2. d, p. 348
3. a, p. 348
4. a, p. 351
5. d, p. 352
6. a, p. 352
7. f, p. 350
8. t, p. 351
9. t, p. 351
10. f, p. 352
11. t, p. 352

How Muscles Are Named
12. c, p. 357
13. a, p. 356
14. f, p. 357
15. e, p. 357
16. g, p. 357
17. b, p. 356
18. d, p. 357

Important Skeletal Muscles: Muscles of the Face and Neck
19. b, p. 358
20. e, p. 358
21. a, p. 358
22. c, p. 358
23. f, p. 362
24. d, p. 358

Important Skeletal Muscles: Trunk Muscles
25. t, p. 366
26. t, p. 366
27. f, p. 370
28. t, p. 363
29. t, p. 356

Important Skeletal Muscles: Upper Limb Muscles
30. a, p. 370
31. c, p. 370
32. a, p. 376
33. d, p. 376
34. f, p. 372
35. t, p. 374
36. t, p. 360
37. t, p. 356
38. f, p. 376

Important Skeletal Muscles: Lower Limb Muscles
39. d, p. 385
40. a, p. 385
41. c, p. 388
42. d, p. 386
43. a, p. 385
44. t, p. 383
45. f, p. 381
46. f, p. 385

Applying What You Know
47. (a) Carpal tunnel syndrome
    (b) The wrist, hand, and fingers are affected due to tenosynovitis. Pain may radiate to the forearm and shoulder.
    (c) Injections of anti-inflammatory agents or surgical removal of tissue pressing on median nerve.
48. deltoid area
49. See tables 10-2 and 10-7 to 10-18

One Last Quick Check
50. c, a, b, pp. 356 and 370
51. a, p. 386
52. a, b, pp. 363 and 386
53. a, p. 376
54. c, p. 381
55. b, f, p. 356
56. a, p. 381
57. a, d, p. 356
58. b, p. 356
59. b, p. 376
60. a, p. 362
61. b, p. 356
62. d, a, p. 381
63. d, p. 350
64. b, p. 350
65. a, p. 351
66. e, p. 351
67. c, p. 351

Diagrams

Facial Muscles Lateral View
1. temporalis
2. masseter
3. sternocleidomastoid
4. orbicularis oris
5. buccinator
6. zygomaticus major
7. orbicularis oculi (palpebral portion)
8. orbicularis oculi
9. corrugator supercilii
10. occipitofrontalis (frontal portion)

Anterior View
1. occipitofrontalis (frontal portion)
2. orbicularis oculi
3. orbicularis oculi (palpebral portion)
4. orbicularis oris
5. buccinator
6. masseter
7. corrugator supercilii
8. temporalis

Muscles of the Thorax
1. external intercostals
2. diaphragm
3. central tendon of diaphragm
4. internal intercostals

Muscles of the Trunk and Abdominal Wall
1. rectus abdominis
2. rectus abdominis (covered by sheath)
3. external abdominal oblique

4. inguinal ligament
5. internal abdominal oblique
6. transverse abdominus
7. linea alba

Muscles Acting on the Shoulder Girdle

1. trapezius
2. seventh cervical vertebra
3. rhomboideus major
4. rhomboideus minor
5. levator scapulae
6. pectoralis minor (cut)
7. subscapularis
8. latissimus dorsi
9. serratus anterior
10. latissimus dorsi (cut)
11. pectoralis minor
12. teres major
13. teres minor
14. subscapularis

Rotator Cuff Muscles

1. clavicle
2. acromion process
3. infraspinatus
4. greater tubercle
5. teres minor
6. intertubercular (bicipital) groove
7. humerus
8. subscapularis
9. lesser tubercle
10. supraspinatus
11. coracoid process

Muscles that Move the Upper Arm

1. deltoideus (cut)
2. coracobrachialis
3. pectoralis major
4. serratus anterior
5. deltoideus
6. thoracolumbar fascia
7. latissimus dorsi
8. teres major
9. infraspinatus
10. rhomboideus major
11. teres minor
12. rhomboideus minor
13. supraspinatus
14. levator scapulae

Muscles of the Upper Arm

1. triceps brachii
2. brachioradialis
3. brachialis
4. biceps brachii (long head)
5. pectoralis major
6. deltoid
7. clavicle
8. biceps brachii
9. radius
10. pronator teres
11. ulna
12. brachialis
13. triceps brachii
14. teres major
15. coracobrachialis

Muscles that Act on the Forearm

1. coracoid process
2. supraglenoid tuberosity
3. tubercle of radius
4. biceps brachii (short head)
5. biceps brachii (long head)
6. olecranon process of ulna
7. triceps brachii (medial head)
8. triceps brachii: lateral (short head)
9. triceps brachii (long head)
10. posterior surface of humerus; lateral intermuscular septum
11. infraglenoid tubercle
12. coracoid process
13. coracobrachialis
14. medial surface of humerus
15. medial epicondyle of humerus
16. pronator teres
17. lateral surface of radius
18. coronoid process of ulna
19. brachialis
20. humerus (distal half)

Muscles of the Forearm

1. pronator teres
2. palmaris longus
3. flexor pollicis brevis
4. opponens pollicis
5. flexor digiti minimi
6. abductor digiti minimi
7. flexor carpi ulnaris
8. flexor carpi radialis
9. palmar interosseus
10. pronator quadratus
11. flexor digitorum profundus
12. supinator
13. brachioradialis
14. flexor digitorum superficialis
15. extensor carpi ulnaris
16. extensor pollicis brevis
17. extensor pollicis longus
18. abductor pollicis longus
19. extensor carpi radialis brevis
20. extensor carpi radialis longus
21. supinator (deep)

Muscles of the Upper Leg

1. tensor fasciae latae
2. iliotibial tract
3. vastus lateralis
4. vastus medialis
5. rectus femoris
6. sartorius
7. gracilis
8. iliopsoas
9. adductor brevis
10. adductor longus
11. adductor magnus
12. fibula
13. tibia
14. pectineus

Muscles of the Lower Leg

1. soleus
2. extensor digitorum longus
3. peroneus brevis
4. tibialis anterior
5. tibia
6. gastrocnemius
7. calcaneal tendon (Achilles tendon)
8. calcaneus

CHAPTER 11

Function of Skeletal Muscle Tissue

1. b, p. 396
2. a, p. 396
3. a, p. 397
4. d, p. 396
5. c, p. 398
6. a, p. 398
7. c, p. 396
8. a, p. 400
9. c, p. 402
10. b, p. 400
11. t, p. 398
12. f, p. 396
13. f, p. 396
14. t, p. 398
15. t, p. 399
16. t, p. 405
17. f, p. 396
18. f, p. 405
19. t, p. 404
20. t, p. 405

Function of Skeletal Muscle Organs
21. d, p. 408
22. d, p. 409
23. a, p. 408
24. d, p. 415
25. a, p. 410
26. c, p. 412
27. c, p. 412
28. f, p. 406
29. t, p. 414
30. t, p. 409
31. f, p. 411

Function of Cardiac and Smooth Muscle Tissue
32. c, p. 417
33. b, p. 415
34. b, p. 415
35. c, p. 415
36. a, p. 415
37. c, p. 415
38. a, p. 417
39. b, p. 415
40. a, p. 415
41. c, p. 417

Mechanisms of Disease
42. myalgia, p. 419
43. myoglobin, p. 419
44. poliomyelitis, p. 420
45. muscular dystrophy, p. 420
46. myasthenia gravis, p. 420

Applying What You Know
47. Linda may have more slow and intermediate fibers than fast fibers. The former are conducive to long races rather than short ones.
48. Muscles in a dead body may be stiff because individual muscle fibers ran out of the ATP required to "turn off" a muscle contraction.

One Last Quick Check
49. a, p. 415
50. b, p. 415
51. b, p. 412
52. d, p. 402
53. a, p. 415
54. d, p. 409
55. f, p. 404
56. t, p. 408
57. t, p. 410
58. t, p. 409
59. t, p. 420
60. t, p. 417
61. t, p. 415
62. t, p. 411
63. f, p. 405

Diagrams

Structure of Skeletal Muscle
1. muscle
2. fascia
3. tendon
4. bone
5. sarcoplasmic reticulum
6. T tubule
7. sarcomere
8. thick filament
9. Z disk
10. thin filament
11. Z line
12. myofibril
13. muscle fiber
14. fascicle

15. endomysium
16. perimysium
17. epimysium

Neuromuscular Junction and Skeletal Muscle Cell
1. motor neuron fiber
2. Schwann cell
3. sarcoplasm
4. acetylcholine receptor sites
5. synaptic cleft
6. motor endplate
7. synaptic vesicles
8. myelin sheath
9. sarcomere
10. sarcolemma
11. mitochondria
12. T tubule
13. sarcoplasmic reticulum
14. triad
15. myofibril

Motor Unit
1. myelin sheath
2. Schwann cell
3. neuromuscular junction
4. nucleus
5. muscle fibers
6. myofibrils
7. motor neuron

Cardiac Muscle Fiber
1. intercalated disks
2. sarcomere
3. sarcolemma
4. myofibril
5. mitochondrion
6. sarcoplasmic reticulum
7. T tubule
8. diad
9. nucleus

CHAPTER 12

Organization of the Nervous System
1. c, p. 432
2. f, p. 432
3. a, p. 432
4. h, p. 433
5. g, p. 433

6. b, p. 433
7. d, p. 432
8. e, p. 433

Cells of the Nervous System
9. b, p. 434
10. a, p. 434
11. d, p. 434
12. a, p. 434
13. c, p. 434
14. d, p. 434
15. a, p. 434
16. c, p. 437
17. c, p. 438
18. b, p. 439
19. a, p. 439
20. c, p. 439
21. d, p. 442

Nerves and Tracts
22. c, p. 443
23. b, p. 443
24. b, p. 443
25. d, p. 443
26. c, p. 443

Repair of Nerve Fibers
27. f, p. 443
28. t, p. 443
29. f, p. 444

Nerve Impulses
30. a, p. 444
31. b, p. 444
32. b, p. 444
33. a, p. 446
34. t, p. 444
35. f, p. 447
36. f, p. 445

Action Potential
37. b, p. 449
38. b, p. 447
39. c, p. 449
40. b, p. 449
41. t, p. 447
42. f, p. 448
43. t, p. 448
44. t, p. 456

Synaptic Transmission
45. c, p. 451

46. b, p. 451
47. a, p. 452
48. f, p. 450
49. t, p. 452
50. t, p. 452

Neurotransmitters
51. d, p. 456
52. b, p. 457
53. c, p. 457
54. c, p. 461
55. d, p. 457
56. f, p. 459
57. t, p. 461

Mechanisms of Disease
58. multiple sclerosis
59. glioma
60. glioblastoma multiforme
61. multiple neurofibromato-
    sis
62. glia

Applying What You Know
63. (a) Multiple sclerosis
    (b) CNS (c) Myelin loss
    and demyelination of the
    white matter in the CNS
    (d) No known cure
    (e) Cause is thought to be
    related to autoimmunity
    and viral infections.
64. CNS damage is most
    often permanent. Since
    the damage is suspected
    to involve the spinal
    cord—which is part of the
    CNS—the prognosis for
    repair is not good.

One Last Quick Check
65. presynaptic, p. 451
66. neurotransmitter, p. 457
67. communicate, p. 456
68. specifically, p. 456
69. pain, p. 461
70. sensory, p. 439
71. ganglion, p. 443
72. telodendria, p. 439
73. a, p. 438
74. b, p. 433
75. b, p. 434

76. a, p. 439
77. a, p. 433
78. b, p. 434
79. b, p. 434
80. a, p. 439
81. b, p. 437
82. a, p. 439

Diagrams

Typical Neuron
1. dendrite
2. Golgi apparatus
3. mitochondrion
4. cell body
5. nucleus
6. Nissl bodies
7. axon hillock
8. axon
9. Schwann cell
10. myelin sheath
11. axon collateral
12. node of Ranvier
13. telodendria
14. synaptic knobs

Myelinated Axon
1. node of Ranvier
2. neurilemma
3. neurofibrils
4. plasma membrane of
    axon
5. myelin sheath
6. nucleus of Schwann cell

Classification of Neurons
1. multipolar neuron
2. bipolar neuron
3. unipolar neuron

Reflex Arc
1. gray matter
2. interneuron
3. sensory neuron axon
4. cell body
5. spinal nerve
6. motor neuron axon
7. white matter
8. dendrite
9. synapse

Chemical Synapse
1. voltage-gated Ca^{++} chan-
    nels

2. synaptic cleft
3. stimulus-gated Na$^+$ channels
4. presynaptic cell
5. postsynaptic cell
6. action potential
7. voltage-gated K$^+$ channels
8. synaptic knob

CHAPTER 13

Coverings of the Brain and Spinal Cord
1. a, p. 472
2. c, p. 472
3. b, p. 474
4. c, p. 472

Cerebrospinal Fluid
5. c, p. 475
6. a, p. 475
7. d, p. 475
8. d, p. 474
9. t, p. 475
10. f, p. 477

The Spinal Cord
11. b, p. 479
12. d, p. 480
13. a, p. 479
14. c, p. 480
15. b, p. 480
16. d, p. 480
17. c, p. 480
18. a, p. 480
19. e, p. 480

The Brain
20. b, p. 482
21. d, p. 484
22. a, p. 485
23. b, p. 488
24. d, p. 489
25. c, p. 490
26. b, p. 496
27. a, p. 490
28. b, p. 498
29. a, p. 497
30. t, p. 484
31. f, p. 487

32. f, p. 484
33. t, p. 490
34. t, p. 490

Somatic Sensory and Motor Pathways
35. c, p. 501
36. c, p. 502
37. a, p. 504
38. t, p. 502
39. f, p. 503

Mechanisms of Disease
40. d, p. 505
41. b, p. 505
42. a, p. 505
43. c, p. 506

Applying What You Know
44. hydrocephalus
45. (a) dementia
    (b) Alzheimer disease

One Last Quick Check
46. h, p. 505
47. d, p. 505
48. e, p. 505
49. c, p. 500
50. j, p. 500
51. a, p. 500
52. b, p. 500
53. f, p. 494
54. i, p. 505
55. g, p. 505
56. e, p. 483
57. d, p. 484
58. a, p. 487
59. d, p. 487
60. e, p. 495
61. b, p. 494
62. c, p. 494
63. d, p. 498
64. c, p. 490
65. d, p. 497
66. d, p. 493

Diagrams

Coverings of the Brain
1. superior sagittal sinus (of dura)
2. subdural space
3. skull

4. falx cerebri
5. muscle
6. skin
7. subarachnoid space
8. arachnoid
9. periosteum
10. epidural space

Fluid Spaces of the Brain
1. cerebral hemisphere
2. anterior horn of lateral ventricle
3. interventricular foramen
4. third ventricle
5. inferior horn of lateral ventricle
6. fourth ventricle
7. pons
8. central canal of spinal cord
9. cerebellum
10. cerebral aqueduct
11. posterior horn of lateral ventricle

Flow of Cerebrospinal Fluid and the Layers of the Brain
1. arachnoid villus
2. choroid plexus of lateral ventricle
3. superior sagittal sinus
4. interventricular foramen
5. choroid plexus of third ventricle
6. cerebral aqueduct
7. choroid plexus of fourth ventricle
8. median foramen
9. central canal of spinal cord
10. dura mater
11. cisterna magna
12. lateral foramen
13. cerebral cortex
14. subarachnoid space
15. arachnoid layer
16. falx cerebri
17. pia mater

Spinal Cord
1. anterior median fissure
2. posterior column
3. gray matter

4. central canal
5. dorsal nerve root
6. spinal nerve
7. lateral column
8. anterior column
9. white matter
10. end of spinal column
11. filum terminale
12. cauda equina
13. lumbar enlargement
14. cervical enlargement

Spinal Cord Tracts
1. fasciculus cuneatus
2. posterior spinocerebellar
3. lateral spinothalamic
4. anterior spinocerebellar
5. spinotectal
6. anterior spinothalamic
7. tectospinal
8. vestibulospinal
9. recticulospinal
10. anterior corticospinal
11. rubrospinal
12. lateral corticospinal
13. fasciculus gracilis

Left Hemisphere of Cerebrum
1. central sulcus
2. superior frontal gyrus
3. frontal lobe
4. lateral fissure
5. temporal lobe
6. occipital lobe
7. parietooccipital fissure
8. parietal lobe
9. postcentral gyrus

Cerebral Cortex
1. precentral gyrus
2. premotor area
3. prefrontal area
4. Broca's area
5. transverse gyrus
6. auditory association area
7. primary auditory area
8. Wernicke's area
9. visual cortex
10. visual association area
11. somatic sensory association area

12. primary taste area
13. postcentral gyrus

CHAPTER 14

Spinal Nerves
1. a, p. 516
2. c, p. 516
3. a, p. 516
4. b, p. 518
5. a, p. 520
6. t, p. 516
7. t, p. 516
8. f, p. 523
9. f, p. 523
10. t, p. 520

Cranial Nerves
11. g, p. 525
12. a, p. 525
13. j, p. 529
14. h, p. 530
15. b, p. 525
16. e, p. 525
17. i, p. 528
18. c, p. 525
19. d, p. 525
20. f, p. 525
21. l, p. 532
22. k, p. 529

Somatic Motor Nervous System
23. b, p. 533
24. a, p. 534
25. a, p. 533

Autonomic Nervous System
26. c, p. 535
27. d, p. 536
28. b, p. 540
29. a, p. 543
30. b, p. 543
31. f, p. 535
32. t, p. 535
33. t, p. 536
34. f, p. 544
35. t, p. 544

Applying What You Know
36. (1) Sympathetic
    (2a) Muscular—skeletal muscles faster
    (2b) Circulatory—stronger heartbeat, dilated blood vessels
    (2c) Respiratory—dilated bronchi
    (2d) Digestive—increased blood sugar levels
    (3) Dysfunction of the sympathetic effectors and perhaps even the ANS itself.
37. (a) Herpes zoster or shingles
    (b) Varicella zoster virus of chickenpox
    (c) It attacks a dermatome (T-4) and symptoms occur in that region.
    (d) His immunological protective mechanism may have become diminished due to the stress.

One Last Quick Check
38. d, p. 535
39. e, p. 535
40. f, p. 535
41. b, p. 535
42. a, p. 535
43. c, p. 533
44. c, p. 536
45. b, p. 536
46. b, p. 539
47. d, p. 539
48. b, p. 543
49. a, p. 543
50. a, p. 543
51. b, p. 543
52. a, p. 543
53. b, p. 543
54. a, p. 543
55. a, p. 543
56. b, p. 543
57. b, p. 543
58. a, p. 523
59. b, p. 523
60. a, p. 532
61. b, p. 523

62. b, p. 516
63. a, p. 525
64. b, p. 516
65. b, p. 518

Diagrams

Spinal Nerves
1. cervical vertebrae
2. brachial plexus
3. thoracic vertebrae
4. lumbar vertebrae
5. sacrum
6. coccyx
7. cervical plexus
8. cervical nerves
9. thoracic nerves
10. dura mater
11. cauda equina
12. lumbar nerves
13. sacral nerves
14. coccygeal nerve

Cranial Nerves
1. trochlear nerve
2. optic nerve
3. oculomotor nerve
4. abducens nerve
5. facial nerve
6. vestibulocochlear nerve
7. vagus nerve
8. accessory nerve
9. hypoglossal nerve
10. glossopharyngeal nerve
11. trigeminal nerve
12. olfactory nerve

Patellar Reflex
1. gray matter
2. spinal cord
3. motor neuron
4. quadriceps muscle
5. patellar tendon
6. patella
7. stretch receptor
8. sensory neuron
9. dorsal root ganglion
10. interneuron

Autonomic Conduction Path
1. somatic motor neuron axon
2. collateral ganglion
3. postganglionic neuron axon
4. sympathetic ganglion
5. preganglionic sympathetic neuron axon

CHAPTER 15

Sensory Receptors
1. b, p. 554
2. d, p. 555
3. a, p. 558
4. b, p. 556
5. a, p. 555
6. f, p. 555
7. t, p. 557
8. f, p. 555
9. t, p. 560
10. t, p. 554

The Sense of Smell and the Sense of Taste
11. b, p. 560
12. d, p. 560
13. c, p. 563
14. b, p. 563
15. t, p. 560
16. f, p. 560
17. t, p. 561
18. f, p. 562

Sense of Hearing and Balance: The Ear
19. a, p. 564
20. c, p. 564
21. d, p. 566
22. d, p. 565
23. b, p. 569
24. b, p. 567
25. a, p. 563
26. t, p. 565
27. f, p. 564
28. t, p. 566
29. t, p. 566
30. f, p. 570

Vision: The Eye
31. c, p. 571
32. a, p. 571
33. a, p. 572
34. d, p. 573
35. d, p. 573
36. a, p. 571
37. c, p. 576
38. a, p. 576
39. c, p. 577
40. a, p. 574
41. f, p. 573
42. f, p. 574
43. t, p. 582
44. t, p. 575
45. f, p. 579
46. t, p. 578
47. t, p. 572
48. t, p. 576
49. f, p. 577
50. f, p. 577

Mechanisms of Disease
51. c, p. 580
52. a, p. 580
53. d, p. 580
54. e, p. 581
55. b, p. 580
56. f, p. 581
57. c, p. 582
58. e, p. 582
59. f, p. 582
60. a, p. 582
61. j, p. 582
62. b, p. 582
63. h, p. 582
64. g, p. 583
65. i, p. 584
66. d, p. 583

Applying What You Know
67. The eustachian tube connects the throat to the middle ear and provides a perfect pathway for the spread of infection.
68. (a) Legally blind (b) 20/200 (c) myopia (d) concave contact lenses or glasses

One Last Quick Check
69. a, p. 565
70. b, p. 566
71. a, p. 564
72. c, p. 570
73. b, p. 571
74. b, p. 559

75. d, p. 573
76. b, p. 574
77. d, p. 562
78. a, p. 563
79. t, p. 564
80. f, p. 583
81. t, p. 582
82. f, p. 569
83. t, p. 582
84. t, p. 576
85. t, p. 572
86. t, p. 555
87. t, p. 559
88. t, p. 568

Diagrams

Midsagittal Section of the Nasal Area
1. olfactory bulb
2. fibers of olfactory nerve
3. cribriform plate of ethmoid bone
4. olfactory tract
5. olfactory recess
6. nasopharynx
7. palate
8. nasal cavity
9. frontal bone

The Ear
1. auricle
2. temporal bone
3. external auditory meatus
4. tympanic membrane
5. semicircular canals
6. oval window
7. facial nerve
8. vestibular nerve
9. cochlear nerve
10. cochlea
11. vestibule
12. round window
13. auditory tube
14. stapes
15. incus
16. malleus

The Eye
1. lens
2. pupil
3. lacrimal caruncle
4. optic disk
5. optic nerve
6. central artery and vein
7. fovea
8. macula lutea
9. posterior chamber
10. sclera
11. choroid
12. retina
13. ciliary body
14. lower lid
15. iris
16. anterior chamber
17. cornea

Extrinsic Muscles of the Right Eye
1. superior oblique
2. medial rectus
3. superior rectus
4. optic nerve
5. levator palpebrae superioris (cut)
6. lateral rectus
7. inferior oblique
8. trochlea

Lacrimal Apparatus
1. caruncle
2. lacrimal canals
3. lacrimal sac
4. nasolacrimal duct
5. puncta
6. lacrimal ducts
7. lacrimal gland

CHAPTER 16

The Endocrine System and Hormones
1. a, p. 594
2. c, p. 594
3. d, p. 595
4. c, p. 594
5. a, p. 595
6. d, p. 597
7. c, p. 595
8. a, p. 601
9. c, p. 602
10. b, p. 599
11. t, p. 594
12. t, p. 595
13. f, p. 599
14. f, p. 604
15. t, p. 594

Prostaglandins
16. b, p. 604
17. c, p. 606

Pituitary Gland
18. b, p. 607
19. a, p. 609
20. d, p. 612
21. c, p. 608
22. b, p. 612
23. a, p. 608
24. d, p. 610
25. c, p. 609
26. e, p. 610
27. h, p. 610
28. g, p. 610
29. f, p. 608
30. i, p. 608
31. b, p. 612

Pineal, Thyroid, and Parathyroid Glands
32. b, p. 615
33. b, p. 614
34. b, p. 614
35. b, p. 618
36. c, p. 618
37. t, p. 616
38. f, p. 617
39. t, p. 616
40. t, p. 613
41. f, p. 614

Adrenal Glands
42. b, p. 619
43. d, p. 619
44. a, p. 621
45. t, p. 619
46. f, p. 623
47. t, p. 621

Pancreatic Islets
48. c, p. 625
49. a, p. 626
50. t, p. 626
51. f, p. 625
52. b, p. 625
53. c, p. 625
54. a, p. 625

55. d, p. 625

Other Endocrine Glands and Tissues
56. a, p. 631
57. b, p. 631
58. c, p. 631
59. f, p. 631
60. t, p. 632
61. t, p. 631

Mechanisms of Disease
62. e, p. 633
63. h, p. 633
64. a, p. 633
65. c, p. 634
66. f, p. 634
67. g, p. 634
68. b, p. 634
69. d, p. 634

Applying What You Know
70. (a) hCG is high during early pregnancy (b) placenta (c) It forms on the lining of the uterus as an interface between the circulatory systems of the mother and the developing child. It is a temporary endocrine gland.
71. (a) Diabetes mellitus (b) inadequate amount or abnormal type of insulin (c) insulin
72. oxytocin

One Last Quick Check
73. a, p. 619
74. c, p. 634
75. d, p. 616
76. c, p. 608
77. d, p. 631
78. d, p. 612
79. b, p. 631
80. d, p. 622
81. d, p. 625
82. b, p. 604
83. j, p. 634
84. g, p. 631
85. h, p. 634
86. i, p. 608

87. b, p. 634
88. f, p. 631
89. a, p. 633
90. d, p. 613
91. e, p. 633
92. c, p. 621

Diagrams
Major Endocrine Glands
1. pineal
2. parathyroids
3. testes (male)
4. ovaries (female)
5. pancreas (islets)
6. adrenals
7. thymus
8. thyroid
9. pituitary
10. hypothalamus

Location and Structure of Pituitary Gland
1. optic chiasma
2. infundibulum
3. pituitary diaphragm
4. pituitary gland
5. nasal cavity
6. brainstem
7. hypothalamus
8. pineal gland
9. thalamus
10. pars anterior
11. pars intermedia
12. adenohypophysis
13. sphenoid bone
14. neurohypophysis
15. infundibulum
16. mammillary body
17. third ventricle
18. optic chiasma

Structure of Thyroid and Parathyroid Glands
1. epiglottis
2. hyoid bone
3. larynx
4. superior parathyroid gland
5. thyroid gland
6. inferior parathyroid glands
7. trachea

CHAPTER 17

Composition of Blood and Red Blood Cells
1. a, p. 648
2. a, p. 649
3. c, p. 649
4. b, p. 650
5. d, p. 652
6. t, p. 649
7. f, p. 651
8. t, p. 651
9. f, p. 653
10. f, p. 651

White Blood Cells and Platelets
11. d, p. 655
12. i, p. 655
13. b, p. 655
14. c, p. 655
15. f, p. 655
16. h, p. 656
17. j, p. 657
18. g, p. 658
19. a, p. 655
20. e, p. 655

Blood Types
21. b, p. 658
22. a, p. 659
23. a, p. 659
24. t, p. 659
25. f, p. 659
26. f, p. 659

Blood Plasma
27. t, p. 662
28. t, p. 662
29. f, p. 662

Blood Clotting
30. b, p. 662
31. d, p. 665
32. c, p. 665

Mechanisms of Disease
33. Polycythemia
34. Aplastic anemia
35. pernicious anemia

36. sickle cell anemia
37. Leukopenia
38. thrombus
39. embolus
40. Hemophilia

Applying What You Know

41. Theoretically, infused red blood cells and elevation of hemoglobin levels after transfusion should increase oxygen consumption and muscle performance during exercise. In practice, however, the advantage appears to be minimal.
42. No. If Mrs. Shearer were a negative Rh factor and her husband were a positive Rh factor, it would set up the strong possibility of erythroblastosis fetalis.
43. Both procedures assist the clotting process.

One Last Quick Check

44. b, p. 668
45. b, p. 667
46. a, p. 655
47. a, p. 662
48. d, p. 660
49. a, p. 655
50. a, p. 671
51. d, p. 659
52. c, p. 650
53. b, p. 663
54. d, p. 655
55. f, p. 667
56. h, p. 658
57. a, p. 655
58. g, p. 668
59. c, p. 657
60. b, p. 659
61. e, p. 660
62. i, p. 659
63. j, p. 655
64. l, p. 657
65. k, p. 649

Diagram

1. basophil

2. neutrophil
3. eosinophil
4. lymphocyte
5. monocyte

CHAPTER 18

Heart

1. b, p. 678
2. c, p. 682
3. a, p. 684
4. a, p. 684
5. d, p. 685
6. d, p. 687
7. c, p. 687
8. d, p. 683
9. d, p. 685
10. b, p. 690
11. Trace the Blood Flow, p. 684 tricuspid (3) pulmonary arteries (6) bicuspid (9) vena cava (1) right ventricle (4) aorta (12) pulmonary semilunar valve (5) left ventricle (10) right atrium (2) left atrium (8) aortic semilunar valve (11)
12. echocardiography, p. 688
13. cardiac enzyme studies, p. 689
14. cardiac nuclear scanning, p. 691
15. cardiopulmonary resuscitation (CPR), p. 678

Blood Vessels

16. d, p. 692
17. c, p. 692
18. e, p. 695
19. g, p. 695
20. f, p. 692
21. b, p. 692
22. a, p. 692
23. t, p. 694
24. f, p. 695
25. t, p. 692
26. f, p. 692

Major Blood Vessels

27. d, p. 696

28. c, p. 696
29. b, p. 696
30. d, p. 706
31. b, p. 714
32. b, p. 714
33. a, p. 714
34. d, p. 696
35. systemic circulation, p. 696
36. circle of Willis, p. 699
37. veins, p. 704
38. hepatic portal system, p. 714
39. ascites, p. 707
40. (a) umbilical arteries (b) umbilical veins, p. 714
41. veins, p. 704

Mechanisms of Disease

42. i, p. 719
43. b, p. 721
44. d, p. 721
45. c, p. 721
46. a, p. 719
47. c, p. 722
48. f, p. 724
49. g, p. 724
50. j, p. 724
51. h, p. 722
52. l, p. 718
53. k, p. 718

Applying What You know

54. Congestive heart failure. Left-sided heart failure often leads to right-sided heart failure. The combination of both problems may require a transplant, implant, or may lead to death.
55. coronary bypass surgery
56. Cardiac enzymes usually increase over the next few hours following a heart attack. These elevations suggest that Mr. Wertz may have had a myocardial infarction with resulting heart muscle damage.

One Last Quick Check

57. c, p. 685
58. d, p. 718
59. c, p. 678
60. d, p. 685
61. b, p. 724
62. b, p. 721
63. g, p. 699
64. a, p. 721
65. i, p. 707
66. c, p. 714
67. f, p. 721
68. b, p. 724
69. h, p. 696
70. d, p. 722
71. e, p. 696
72. j, p. 719

Diagrams

Heart
1. aorta
2. superior vena cava
3. right atrium
4. left AV (mitral or bicus-pid) valve
5. right AV (tricuspid) valve
6. chordae tendineae
7. right ventricle
8. interventricular septum
9. papillary muscle
10. left ventricle
11. right ventricle
12. pulmonary veins
13. right atrium
14. openings of coronary arteries
15. pulmonary trunk
16. aortic semilunar valve
17. left atrium

Blood Vessels
1. tunica adventitia
2. tunica media
3. tunica intima
4. tunica adventitia
5. tunica media
6. tunica intima

Veins
1. facial
2. right brachiocephalic
3. right subclavian
4. superior vena cava
5. inferior vena cava
6. hepatic
7. hepatic portal
8. median cubital
9. superior mesenteric
10. common iliac
11. external iliac
12. femoral
13. great saphenous
14. small saphenous
15. dorsal venous arch
16. digital
17. posterior tibial
18. anterior tibial
19. fibular
20. popliteal
21. femoral
22. digital
23. internal iliac
24. common iliac
25. inferior mesenteric
26. splenic
27. median basilic
28. basilic
29. axillary
30. cephalic
31. internal jugular
32. external jugular
33. superior sagittal sinus

Arteries
1. right common carotid
2. brachiocephalic
3. axillary
4. brachial
5. superior mesenteric
6. abdominal aorta
7. common iliac
8. internal iliac
9. external iliac
10. deep medial circumflex femoral
11. deep femoral
12. femoral
13. popliteal
14. anterior tibial
15. peroneal
16. posterior tibial
17. arcuate
18. dorsal metatarsal
19. dorsal pedis
20. digital
21. palmar arch
22. ulnar
23. radial
24. arch of aorta
25. left subclavian
26. external carotid
27. internal carotid

Fetal Circulation
1. superior vena cava
2. foramen ovale
3. inferior vena cava
4. ductus venosus
5. umbilical vein
6. fetal umbilicus
7. umbilical cord
8. internal iliac arteries
9. common iliac artery
10. pulmonary trunk
11. ductus arteriosus

CHAPTER 19

Hemodynamics and the Heart as a Pump
1. b, p. 737
2. b, p. 735
3. a, p. 738
4. b, p. 738
5. a, p. 743
6. t, p. 742
7. f, p. 770
8. f, p. 770
9. t, p. 770
10. t, p. 742

Circulation and Blood Pressure
11. d, p. 745
12. c, p. 747
13. b, p. 748
14. d, p. 749
15. d, p. 751
16. a, p. 754
17. b, p. 762
18. c, p. 766
19. b, p. 751
20. d, p. 753
21. f, p. 746
22. t, p. 746
23. t, p. 748
24. t, p. 756

25. f, p. 757
26. t, p. 760
27. t, p. 762
28. t, p. 765
29. f, p. 766
30. t, p. 754

Mechanisms of Disease
31. septic shock
32. Cardiogenic shock
33. anaphylaxis; anaphylactic shock
34. Neurogenic shock
35. low blood volume
36. toxic shock syndrome

Applying What You Know
37. (a) Hypovolemic shock (b) The body might respond by increasing the heart rate, decreasing the urine output and decreasing available fluids to the tissues.
38. (a) heart block (b) artificial pacemaker

One Last Quick Check
39. c, p. 769
40. a, p. 772
41. c, p. 772
42. c, p. 755
43. a, p. 772
44. e, p. 734
45. k, p. 735
46. a, p. 738
47. b, p. 770
48. c, p. 770
49. g, p. 742
50. i, p. 742
51. d, p. 748
52. h, p. 754
53. f, p. 754
54. j, p. 763
55. l, p. 766

Diagram

ECG Strip Recording
1. atrial depolarization
2. ventricular depolarization
3. ventricular repolarization

CHAPTER 20

Lymphatic Vessels, Lymph, and Circulation of Lymph
1. c, p. 780
2. b, p. 781
3. a, p. 781
4. d, p. 781
5. c, p. 782
6. b, p. 782
7. a, p. 782
8. t, p. 780
9. f, p. 781
10. t, p. 781
11. f, p. 781
12. t, p. 782
13. t, p. 781
14. t, p. 782

Lymph Nodes
15. b, p. 786
16. d, p. 785
17. a, p. 788
18. c, p. 788
19. f, p. 785
20. t, p. 785

Lymphatic Drainage of the Breast
21. a, p. 789
22. c, p. 788

Tonsils, Thymus, and Spleen
23. a, p. 790
24. c, p. 791
25. c, p. 790
26. f, p. 791
27. f, p. 792
28. t, p. 793

Mechanisms of Disease
29. Lymphoma
30. acute otitis media
31. blood poisoning
32. filaria
33. Hodgkin and non-Hodgkin

Applying What You Know
34. (a) Yes (b) Yes (c) The spleen destroys old blood cells and platelets. Pre-venting this will allow Nancy to preserve her own supply and avoid anemia.
35. Baby Wilson had no means of producing T cells, thus making him susceptible to several diseases. Isolation was a means of controlling his exposure to these diseases.

One Last Quick Check
36. b, p. 790
37. c, p. 792
38. c, p. 793
39. a, p. 790
40. c, p. 793
41. a, p. 791
42. a, p. 790
43. t, p. 781
44. t, p. 782
45. t, p. 785
46. f, p. 785
47. t, p. 794
48. f, p. 789
49. f, p. 792
50. f, p. 793

Diagrams

Principal Organs of the Lymphatic System
1. thymus gland
2. right lymphatic duct
3. thoracic duct
4. intestinal duct
5. appendix
6. bone marrow
7. inguinal lymph nodes
8. Peyer's patches in intestinal wall
9. spleen
10. mammary plexus
11. axillary lymph node
12. cervical lymph node
13. tonsils

Lymph Node
1. afferent lymph vessel
2. capsule
3. trabeculae

4. efferent lymph vessel
5. hilus
6. medullary cords
7. medullary sinus
8. cortical nodules
9. sinuses
10. germinal center

Lymphatic Drainage of Breast
1. supraclavicular nodes
2. midaxillary nodes
3. lateral axillary nodes
4. subscapular nodes
5. anterior axillary (pectoral) nodes
6. internal mammary nodes
7. interpectoral (Rotter) nodes

CHAPTER 21

Innate Immunity
1. d, p. 804
2. c, p. 805
3. a, p. 808
4. a, p. 807
5. b, p. 808
6. f, p. 802
7. t, p. 803
8. f, p. 810
9. f, p. 810
10. t, p. 808

Adaptive Immunity
11. b, p. 811
12. b, p. 811
13. d, p. 811
14. a, p. 815
15. b, p. 819
16. b, p. 816
17. c, p. 814
18. b, p. 821
19. b, p. 817
20. b, p. 821
21. t, p. 816
22. f, p. 816
23. t, p. 819
24. t, p. 819
25. t, p. 825
26. t, p. 823

27. t, p. 823
28. t, p. 822
29. f, p. 824
30. f, p. 819

Mechanisms of Disease
31. f, p. 831
32. t, p. 831
33. t, p. 829
34. f, p. 831
35. f, p. 830

Applying What You Know
36. (a) Passive acquired immunity (b) active artificial immunity (c) Active immunity usually lasts longer than passive.
37. (a) AIDS (b) azidothymidine (AZT) and dideoxyinosine (DDI)

One Last Quick Check
38. a, p. 820
39. d, p. 831
40. b, p. 810
41. d, p. 814
42. b, p. 818
43. d, p. 821
44. c, p. 824
45. c, p. 825
46. a, p. 824
47. b, p. 824
48. d, p. 825

CHAPTER 22

Selye's Concept of Stress
1. b, p. 842
2. b, p. 842
3. b, p. 843
4. b, p. 841
5. d, p. 841
6. f, p. 842
7. f, p. 846
8. t, p. 842
9. f, p. 840
10. t, p. 844

Some Current Concepts About Stress

11. c, p. 845
12. d, p. 845
13. b, p. 847
14. t, p. 844
15. f, p. 846
16. f, p. 847
17. t, p. 845
18. f, p. 847

Applying What You Know
19. (a) Stress (b) See Figure 22-6, page 845 (c) Immune diseases, decreased quality of life, ulcers, hypertension, chemical dependency, impaired relationships, and loss of contact with reality.
20. (a) Sympathetic (b) No, digestion decreases under the influence of the sympathetic nervous system.

One Last Quick Check
21. General adaptation syndrome, p. 840
22. exhaustion, p. 842
23. corticotropin releasing hormone, p. 844
24. fight or flight reaction, p. 845
25. Psychophysiology, p. 847
26. f, p. 846
27. t, p. 840
28. t, p. 846
29. f, p. 848
30. t, p. 842

CHAPTER 23

Upper Respiratory Tract
1. a, p. 856
2. c, p. 856
3. d, p. 858
4. c, p. 858
5. a, p. 861
6. f, p. 857
7. f, p. 860
8. t, p. 860
9. f, p. 861
10. t, p. 861

Lower Respiratory Tract

11. a, p. 862
12. b, p. 867
13. c, p. 870
14. d, p. 871
15. f, p. 862
16. f, p. 862
17. t, p. 864
18. f, p. 869
19. f, p. 869
20. t, p. 867

Mechanisms of Disease

21. d, p. 875
22. g, p. 873
23. b, p. 872
24. a, p. 873
25. c, p. 872
26. f, p. 872
27. e, p. 872
28. h, p. 860

Applying What You Know

29. (a) epiglottis
    (b) *Haemophilus influenzae* type B
    (c) yes
30. (a) croup
    (b) no
31. During the day Mr. Gorski's cilia are paralyzed because of his heavy smoking. They use the time when Mr. Gorski is asleep to sweep accumulations of mucus and bacteria toward the pharynx. When Mr. Gorski awakens, these collections are waiting to be eliminated.

One Last Quick Check

32. a, p. 859
33. b, p. 860
34. a, p. 858
35. a, p. 858
36. a, p. 858
37. b, p. 860
38. b, p. 872
39. c, p. 861
40. a, p. 872
41. b, p. 872
42. a, p. 872
43. air distributor, p. 856
44. gas exchanger, p. 856
45. filters, p. 856
46. warms, p. 856
47. humidifies, p. 856
48. nose, p. 857
49. pharynx, p. 857
50. larynx, p. 857
51. trachea, p. 857
52. bronchi, p. 857
53. lungs, p. 857
54. alveoli, p. 865
55. Exchange, p. 867
56. respiratory membrane, p. 869
57. surface, p. 869

Diagrams

Respiratory System

1. upper respiratory tract
2. lower respiratory tract
3. alveolar duct
4. alveolar sac
5. bronchioles
6. primary bronchi
7. trachea
8. larynx
9. laryngopharynx
10. oropharynx
11. nasopharynx
12. nasal cavity

Nasal Cavity

1. cribriform plate of ethmoid bone
2. frontal sinus
3. superior turbinate
4. middle turbinate
5. inferior turbinate
6. vestibule
7. anterior naris
8. pharyngeal tonsil
9. posterior naris
10. sella turcica
11. sphenoid sinus

Divisions of Pharynx

1. opening of eustachian tube
2. soft palate
3. hyoid bone
4. lingual tonsil
5. vocal cords
6. trachea
7. esophagus
8. laryngopharynx
9. epiglottis
10. oropharynx
11. palatine tonsil
12. uvula
13. nasopharynx
14. pharyngeal tonsil

Paranasal Sinuses

1. sphenoid sinus
2. maxillary sinus
3. lacrimal sac
4. ethmoid air cells
5. superior turbinate
6. middle turbinate
7. inferior turbinate
8. oral cavity
9. maxillary sinus
10. sphenoid sinus
11. frontal sinus
12. ethmoid air cells
13. frontal sinus

Lobes and Fissures of the Lungs

1. superior lobe
2. middle lobe
3. inferior lobe
4. oblique fissure
5. horizontal fissure
6. oblique fissure
7. inferior lobe
8. superior lobe

CHAPTER 24

Pulmonary Ventilation

1. b, p. 884
2. c, p. 884
3. b, p. 890
4. c, p. 894
5. d, p. 896
6. d, p. 898
7. d, p. 899
8. d, p. 899
9. a, p. 884

10. d, p. 886
11. t, p. 886
12. f, p. 895
13. t, p. 894
14. t, p. 898
15. t, p. 894

Pulmonary Gas Exchange
16. a, p. 900
17. d, p. 901
18. c, p. 900
19. a, p. 901
20. t, p. 896
21. t, p. 899
22. f, p. 903
23. t, p. 900

Blood Transportation of Gases and Systemic Gas Exchange
24. d, p. 903
25. b, p. 903
26. d, p. 906
27. c, p. 904
28. t, p. 904
29. f, p. 906
30. f, p. 908
31. t, p. 910

Regulation of Breathing
32. d, p. 912
33. b, p. 914
34. f, p. 912
35. t, p. 914

Mechanisms of Disease
36. COPD; chronic obstructive pulmonary disease
37. Bronchitis
38. Emphysema
39. Asthma

Applying What You Know
40. (a) obstructive pulmonary disorders (b) COPD which may include bronchitis, emphysema, and asthma (c) They obstruct inspiration and expiration. The primary difficulty is in emptying their lungs adequately which

creates a buildup of CO_2 in the lungs.
41. The "diving reflex" was responsible for this phenomenon. It is a protective response of the body to cold water immersion that slows the metabolism and tissue requirements to enable survival.

One Last Quick Check
42. d, p. 884
43. c, p. 906
44. c, p. 903
45. b, p. 892
46. d, p. 897
47. d, p. 894
48. d, p. 895
49. e, p. 894
50. c, p. 897
51. a, p. 896
52. f, p. 897
53. d, p. 899
54. b, p. 903
55. i, p. 898
56. j, p. 912
57. g, p. 912
58. h, p. 912

Diagrams

Pulmonary Volumes
1. total lung capacity (TLC)
2. inspiratory reserve volume (IRV)
3. tidal volume (TV)
4. expiratory reserve volume (ERV)
5. residual volume (RV)
6. vital capacity (VC)

Respiratory Centers of Brainstem
1. limbic system
2. pneumotaxic center
3. respiratory centers
4. apneustic center

5. pons
6. inspiratory center
7. expiratory area
8. medulla
9. respiratory muscles
10. cortex

CHAPTER 25

Overview of the Digestive System
1. c, p. 927
2. b, p. 928
3. t, p. 926
4. f, p. 928
5. a, p. 927
6. a, p. 927
7. a, p. 927
8. b, p. 927
9. b, p. 927
10. b, p. 927
11. b, p. 927
12. b, p. 927
13. a, p. 927
14. a, p. 927

Mouth and Pharynx
15. d, p. 929
16. b, p. 930
17. c, p. 932
18. d, p. 933
19. b, p. 934
20. t, p. 932
21. f, p. 929
22. f, p. 933
23. t, p. 934
24. f, p. 929

Esophagus and Stomach
25. b, p. 934
26. d, p. 936
27. c, p. 937
28. t, p. 936
29. t, p. 936
30. t, p. 937

Small Intestine, Large Intestine, Appendix, and Peritoneum
31. c, p. 939

32. b, p. 939
33. a, p. 942
34. b, p. 943
35. f, p. 940
36. f, p. 942
37. t, p. 942
38. t, p. 942

Liver, Gallbladder, and Pancreas
39. b, p. 944
40. d, p. 946
41. b, p. 946
42. a, p. 946
43. t, p. 944
44. f, p. 946
45. t, p. 949
46. t, p. 947

Mechanisms of Disease
47. d, p. 955
48. g, p. 955
49. f, p. 955
50. e, p. 950
51. i, p. 953
52. a, p. 952
53. h, p. 955
54. b, p. 951
55. c, p. 955
56. k, p. 951
57. j, p. 953

Applying What You Know
58. (a) cholelithiasis (b) jaundice (c) obstruction of the bile flow into the duodenum (d) cholecystectomy or ultrasound lithotripsy
59. pylorospasm

One Last Quick Check
60. d, p. 933
61. d, p. 932
62. c, p. 933
63. d, p. 933
64. d, p. 951
65. a, p. 932
66. c, p. 930
67. b, p. 933
68. c, p. 934
69. c, p. 940
70. a, p. 946

71. b, p. 939
72. d, p. 947
73. c, p. 944
74. f, p. 940
75. f, p. 940
76. t, p. 942
77. t, p. 928
78. t, p. 935
79. t, p. 937
80. t, p. 943
81. t, p. 926
82. f, p. 935

Diagrams

Digestive Organs
1. parotid gland
2. submandibular gland
3. pharynx
4. esophagus
5. liver
6. transverse colon
7. ascending colon
8. ileum
9. cecum
10. vermiform appendix
11. rectum
12. sigmoid colon
13. descending colon
14. stomach
15. sublingual gland
16. tongue

Tooth
1. crown
2. neck
3. root
4. bone
5. cementum
6. peridontal membrane
7. peridontal ligament
8. root canal
9. gingiva (gum)
10. pulp cavity with nerves and vessels
11. dentin
12. enamel
13. cusp

Stomach
1. lower esophageal sphincter
2. esophagus
3. gastroesophageal opening
4. lesser curvature
5. pylorus
6. pyloric sphincter
7. duodenal bulb
8. duodenum
9. rugae
10. greater curvature
11. submucosa
12. mucosa
13. oblique muscle layer
14. circular muscle layer
15. longitudinal muscle layer
16. serosa
17. body
18. fundus

Wall of Small Intestine
1. serosa
2. muscularis
3. longitudinal muscle
4. circular muscle
5. submucosa
6. mucosa
7. plica (fold)
8. mesentery

Divisions of Large Intestine
1. transverse colon
2. hepatic flexure
3. ascending colon
4. cecum
5. rectum
6. superior rectal artery and vein
7. sigmoid colon
8. sigmoid artery and vein
9. inferior mesenteric artery and vein
10. descending colon
11. superior mesenteric artery
12. splenic flexure

Liver
1. inferior vena cava
2. right lobe
3. gallbladder
4. round ligament
5. falciform ligament
6. left lobe
7. left lobe
8. falciform ligament

9. hepatic artery
10. hepatic portal vein
11. common hepatic duct
12. quadrate lobe
13. gallbladder
14. right lobe proper
15. inferior vena cava
16. caudate lobe

Common Bile Duct and Its Tributaries

1. right and left hepatic ducts
2. cystic duct
3. common hepatic duct
4. common bile duct
5. accessory duct of pancreas
6. pancreatic duct

CHAPTER 26

Digestion

1. b, p. 962
2. a, p. 962
3. b, p. 970
4. a, p. 971
5. b, p. 972
6. b, p. 968
7. c, p. 972
8. f, p. 965
9. f, p. 968
10. t, p. 969
11. f, p. 970
12. t, p. 973
13. f, p. 968
14. t, p. 971

Secretion and Control of Digestive Gland Secretion

15. b, p. 974
16. b, p. 974
17. d, p. 976
18. d, p. 978
19. t, p. 975
20. t, p. 978
21. f, p. 978
22. t, p. 974

Absorption and Elimination

23. b, p. 982
24. b, p. 984
25. c, p. 982
26. f, p. 980
27. t, p. 980
28. f, p. 984
29. f, p. 981
30. t, p. 981

Mechanisms of Disease

31. h, p. 986
32. d, p. 986
33. g, p. 986
34. a, p. 986
35. f, p. 986
36. b, p. 986
37. i, p. 986
38. c, p. 987
39. j, p. 987
40. e, p. 987

Applying What You Know

41. (a) pain in the abdomen with possible hemorrhage (b) duodenum or possibly the stomach (c) *Helicobacter pylori* bacterium and hyperacidity (d) drugs that reduce hydrochloric acid formation and antibiotics to kill the bacteria
42. Replacement of fluids should focus on large amounts of cool, diluted, or isotonic fluids.

One Last Quick Check

43. a, p. 972
44. c, p. 967
45. a, p. 968
46. b, p. 986
47. c, p. 977
48. c, p. 973
49. a, p. 973
50. b, p. 977
51. d, p. 973
52. c, p. 973
53. c, p. 968

54. a, p. 976
55. d, p. 962
56. c, p. 968
57. f, p. 968
58. t, p. 969
59. t, p. 978
60. t, p. 982
61. f, p. 986

CHAPTER 27

Overview of Nutrition and Metabolism

1. a, p. 995
2. d, p. 994
3. t, p. 995
4. f, p. 995

Carbohydrates

5. a, p. 997
6. b, p. 997
7. c, p. 997
8. a, p. 997
9. a, p. 998
10. b, p. 998
11. d, p. 1003
12. b, p. 1006
13. t, p. 997
14. t, p. 998
15. f, p. 997
16. f, p. 1003
17. t, p. 1006
18. t, p. 1004
19. f, p. 1004
20. t, p. 1006
21. t, p. 1005
22. f, p. 1007
23. f, p. 997
24. t, p. 998
25. t, p. 1000
26. f, p. 1000
27. f, p. 1005

Lipids

28. a, p. 1008
29. c, p. 1008
30. a, p. 1008
31. c, p. 1010

32. d, p. 1009
33. f, p. 1009
34. t, p. 1009
35. t, p. 1010
36. t, p. 1008
37. t, p. 1009

Proteins
38. b, p. 1011
39. b, p. 1012
40. d, p. 1012
41. f, p. 1011
42. t, p. 1011
43. t, p. 1012
44. f, p. 1012
45. t, p. 1012

Vitamins and Minerals
46. b, p. 1013
47. a, p. 1015
48. c, p. 1017
49. f, p. 1013
50. t, p. 1016
51. t, p. 1016
52. f, p. 1013

Metabolic Rate and Mechanisms for Regulating Food Intake
53. b, p. 1018
54. c, p. 1018
55. c, p. 1021
56. b, p. 1021
57. f, p. 1019
58. t, p. 1021
59. t, p. 1021
60. f, p. 1020
61. f, p. 1018

Mechanisms of Disease
62. b, p. 1023
63. e, p. 1025
64. a, p. 1025
65. f, p. 1025
66. d, p. 1025
67. c, p. 1023
68. g, p. 1025

Applying What You Know
69. weight loss and anorexia nervosa
70. Iron would be the first

mineral of choice. It is found in meat, eggs, vegetables, and legumes. Copper sources which might also help the anemia would be seafood, organ meats, and legumes.

One Last Quick Check
71. b, p. 998
72. a, p. 1002
73. c, p. 1006
74. c, p. 1020
75. b, p. 1020
76. d, p. 997
77. a, p. 997
78. bile (all others refer to carbohydrate metabolism)
79. amino acids (all others refer to fat metabolism)
80. M (all others refer to vitamins)
81. iron (all others refer to protein metabolism)
82. insulin (all others tend to increase blood glucose)
83. folic acid (all others are minerals)
84. ascorbic acid (all others refer to the B-complex vitamins)
85. a, p. 997
86. c, p. 1011
87. d, p. 1013
88. e, p. 1015
89. a, p. 997
90. e, p. 1015
91. a, p. 998
92. b. p. 1008
93. b. p. 1009

CHAPTER 28

Anatomy of the Urinary System
1. d, p. 1043
2. c, p. 1034
3. c, p. 1035
4. b, p. 1041
5. d, p. 1041
6. c, p. 1043

7. c, p. 1042
8. a, p. 1043
9. f, p. 1034
10. f, p. 1035
11. t, p. 1041
12. t, p. 1042
13. f, p. 1035
14. t, p. 1041
15. f, p. 1034

Physiology of the Urinary System
16. b, p. 1045
17. a, p. 1045
18. d, p. 1045
19. a, p. 1047
20. c, p. 1049
21. d, p. 1051
22. c, p. 1057
23. d, p. 1054
24. c, p. 1054
25. t, p. 1045
26. f, p. 1047
27. t, p. 1049
28. t, p. 1045
29. f, p. 1046
30. f, p. 1046
31. t, p. 1052
32. f, p. 1046
33. f, p. 1054
34. f, p. 1054
35. t, p. 1046

Mechanisms of Disease
36. i, p. 1057
37. c, p. 1057
38. f, p. 1060
39. g, p. 1058
40. k, p. 1059
41. a, p. 1059
42. h, p. 1060
43. j, p. 1060
44. b, p. 1057
45. d, p. 1060
46. e, p. 1059
47. l, p. 1059

Applying What You Know
48. Hemorrhage causes a drop in blood pressure, which decreases the urine output and can eventually

lead to kidney failure.

49. Stage I—Often asymptomatic because healthy nephrons compensate for the ones destroyed by disease
Stage 2—Renal insufficiency; BUN increases, polyuria and dehydration may occur
Stage 3—Uremia; high BUN, loss of kidney function, oliguria, edema, hypertension, and eventual death if an artificial kidney or transplant not available.

One Last Quick Check

50. b, p. 1055
51. d, p. 1060
52. a, p. 1051
53. c, p. 1041
54. c, p. 1047
55. b, p. 1041
56. c, p. 1038
57. b, p. 1042
58. a, p. 1034
59. b, p. 1039
60. e, p. 1058
61. c, p. 1057
62. f, p. 1059
63. d, p. 1041
64. j, p. 1057
65. h, p. 1057
66. a, p. 1041
67. g, p. 1059
68. i, p. 1039
69. b, p. 1039
70. k, p. 1060

Diagrams

Kidney

1. interlobular arteries
2. renal column
3. renal sinus
4. hilum
5. renal pelvis
6. renal papilla of pyramid
7. ureter
8. medulla

9. medullary pyramid
10. major calyces
11. minor calyces
12. cortex
13. capsule (fibrous)

Nephron

1. cortical nephron
2. proximal tubule
3. glomerulus
4. distal convoluted tubule
5. collecting tubule
6. vasa recta
7. pyramid (medulla)
8. Henle's loop
9. ascending limb of Henle's loop
10. descending limb of Henle's loop
11. arcuate artery and vein
12. juxtamedullary nephron
13. interlobular artery and vein
14. afferent arteriole
15. efferent arteriole

Male Urinary Bladder

1. ureter
2. opening of ureter
3. rugae
4. prostate
5. external urinary sphincter
6. bulbourethral gland
7. prostatic urethra
8. internal urinary sphincter
9. opening of ureter
10. trigone
11. smooth muscle
12. cut edge of peritoneum

CHAPTER 29

Overview of Fluid and Electrolyte Balance

1. c, p. 1068
2. c, p. 1071
3. a, p. 1071
4. b, p. 1071
5. d, p. 1071
6. d, p. 1072
7. c, p. 1070
8. f, p. 1068

9. t, p. 1069
10. t, p. 1072
11. f, p. 1068
12. t, p. 1074
13. f, p. 1072
14. t, p. 1070

Mechanisms that Maintain Homeostasis of Total Fluid Volume

15. d, p. 1075
16. c, p. 1074
17. f, p. 1074
18. t, p. 1076

Regulation of Water and Electrolyte Levels in Plasma, Interstitial Fluid, and Intracellular Fluid

19. a, p. 1077
20. c, p. 1076
21. c, p. 1077
22. c, p. 1080
23. t, p. 1078
24. f, p. 1078
25. t, p. 1080
26. t, p. 1080

Regulation of Sodium and Potassium Levels in Body Fluids

27. f, p. 1080
28. t, p. 1082
29. t, p. 1082
30. f, p. 1076
31. t, p. 1082

Mechanisms of Disease

32. a, p. 1083
33. d, p. 1084
34. e, p. 1083
35. b, p. 1083
36. c, p. 1083
37. t, p. 1083
38. f, p. 1084
39. t, p. 1083
40. f, p. 1084

Applying What You Know

41. Ms. Titus could not accurately measure water intake created by foods or

catabolism, nor could she measure output created by lungs, skin, or the intestines.
42. Jack's body contained more water. Obese people have a lower water content than slender people.

One Last Quick Check
43. inside
44. extracellular
45. extracellular
46. lower
47. more
48. decreases
49. a, p. 1068
50. d, p. 1068
51. c, p. 1072
52. e, p. 1072
53. d, p. 1083
54. c, p. 1069
55. b, p. 1083
56. d, p. 1072
57. a, pp. 1071 and 1078
58. a, p. 1071
59. d, p. 1073
60. t, p. 1069
61. t, p. 1078
62. t, p. 1080

CHAPTER 30

Mechanisms that Control pH of Body Fluids
1. c, p. 1090
2. a, p. 1090
3. b, p. 1091
4. d, p. 1091
5. c, p. 1092
6. a, p. 1091
7. c, p. 1090
8. t, p. 1090
9. f, p. 1091
10. t, p. 1091
11. f, p. 1090
12. t, p. 1091
13. t, p. 1091

Buffer Mechanisms for Controlling pH of Body Fluids

14. a, p. 1092
15. c, p. 1092
16. t, p. 1094
17. f, p. 1095
18. t, p. 1092
19. f, p. 1094
20. t, p. 1094

Respiratory and Urinary Mechanisms of pH Control
21. d, p. 1095
22. b, p. 1096
23. b, p. 1097
24. a, p. 1097
25. c, p. 1098
26. t, p. 1097
27. f, p. 1097
28. t, p. 1098
29. f, p. 1092
30. t, p. 1097

Mechanisms of Disease
31. f, p. 1100
32. e, p. 1100
33. a, p. 1100
34. b, p. 1101
35. g, p. 1101
36. c, p. 1101
37. d, p. 1101

Applying What You Know
38. Normal saline contains chloride ions, which replace bicarbonate ions and thus relieve the bicarbonate excess that occurs during severe vomiting.
39. Most citrus fruits, although acid tasting, are fully oxidized with the help of buffers during metabolism and have little effect on acid-base balance. Cranberry juice is one of the few exceptions.

One Last Quick Check
40. a, p. 1095
41. c, p. 1095
42. a, p. 1097
43. d, p. 1090

44. a, p. 1095
45. d, p. 1101
46. d, p. 1092
47. a, p. 1092
48. g, p. 1090
49. c, p. 1090
50. h, p. 1091
51. e, p. 1101
52. f, p. 1101
53. a, p. 1100
54. b, p. 1092
55. d, p. 1094

CHAPTER 31

Male Reproductive Organs
1. a, p. 1110
2. b, p. 1110
3. c, p. 1110
4. d, p. 1110
5. c, p. 1111
6. a, p. 1112
7. a, p. 1112
8. c, p. 1113
9. t, p. 1112
10. f, p. 1112
11. f, p. 1115
12. t, p. 1113
13. f, p. 1110
14. f, p. 1110
15. t, p. 1112

Reproductive Ducts and Accessory Reproductive Glands
16. b, p. 1116
17. c, p. 1116
18. a, p. 1118
19. c, p. 1118
20. b, p. 1119
21. t, p. 1116
22. t, p. 1116
23. t, p. 1117
24. t, p. 1119

Supporting Structures, Seminal Fluid, and Male Fertility
25. c, p. 1120
26. b, p. 1120
27. b, p. 1121

28. c, p. 1121
29. f, p. 1120
30. t, p. 1120
31. f, p. 1121

Mechanisms of Disease
32. oligospermia
33. 2 months
34. cryptorchidism
35. benign prostatic hypertrophy
36. Phimosis
37. impotence; erectile dysfunction
38. hydrocele
39. inguinal hernia

Applying What You Know
40. (a) cryptorchidism (b) easily detected by palpation of the scrotum (c) surgery or testosterone injections (d) early detection results in normal testicular and sexual development.
41. (a) hydrocele or inguinal hernia (b) inguinal hernia (c) Swelling of the scrotum occurs when the intestine pushes through the weak area of the abdominal wall that separates the abdominopelvic cavity from the scrotum. (d) external supports or surgical repair

One Last Quick Check
42. b, p. 1120
43. c, p. 1120
44. b, p. 1110
45. c, p. 1111
46. a, p. 1112
47. d, p. 1120
48. d, p. 1112
49. d, p. 1113
50. c, p. 1112
51. c, p. 1112

52. a, p. 1113
53. b, p. 1116
54. h, p. 1120
55. g, p. 1118
56. a, p. 1116
57. f, p. 1118
58. c, p. 1116
59. i, p. 1120
60. e, p. 1120
61. d, p. 1120
62. j, p. 1120

Diagrams

Male Pelvis—Sagittal Section
1. rectum
2. seminal vesicle
3. levator ani muscle
4. ejaculatory duct
5. anus
6. bulbocavernosus muscle
7. glans
8. testis
9. urethra
10. corpus spongiosum
11. corpus cavernosum
12. prostate gland
13. symphysis pubis
14. urinary bladder

Tubules of Testis and Epididymis
1. nerves and blood vessels of spermatic cord
2. ductus (vas) deferens
3. septum
4. lobule
5. tunica albuginea
6. testis
7. seminiferous tubules
8. epididymis

Penis
1. bladder
2. prostate
3. bulb
4. deep artery
5. foreskin (prepuce)
6. external urethral orifice

7. glans penis
8. corpus spongiosum
9. urethra
10. corpus cavernosum
11. opening of Cowper's glands
12. crus penis
13. bulbourethral gland
14. openings of ejaculatory ducts

CHAPTER 32

Overview of the Female Reproductive System
1. a, p. 1130
2. b, p. 1130
3. t, p. 1130
4. t, p. 1130

Internal Female Genitals
5. b, p. 1130
6. d, p. 1133
7. b, p. 1134
8. a, p. 1134
9. b, p. 1134
10. d, p. 1136
11. a, p. 1136
12. b, p. 1134
13. c, p. 1138
14. b, p. 1135
15. a, p. 1136
16. b, p. 1134
17. a, p. 1136
18. a, p. 1136
19. c, p. 1138
20. t, p. 1132
21. f, p. 1134
22. f, p. 1134
23. t, p. 1138

External Female Genitals and Breasts
24. c, p. 1138
25. b, p. 1138
26. a, p. 1138
27. a, p. 1140
28. f, p. 1138

29. f, p. 1139
30. f, p. 1140
31. t, p. 1140
32. f, p. 1141

Female Reproductive Cycle
33. a, p. 1141
34. c, p. 1142
35. d, p. 1147
36. c, p. 1143
37. b, p. 1147
38. f, p. 1142
39. t, p. 1143
40. t, p. 1148
41. f, p. 1141
42. f, p. 1143

Mechanisms of Disease
43. f, p. 1152
44. e, p. 1152
45. a, p. 1149
46. h, p. 1152
47. i, p. 1151
48. g, p. 1150
49. c, p. 1150
50. b, p. 1149
51. l, p. 1151
52. d, p. 1149
53. j, p. 1154
54. k, p. 1151

Applying What You Know
55. (a) Contraceptive pills contain synthetic progesterone-like compounds such as progestin, sometimes combined with synthetic estrogens. By sustaining a high blood concentration of these substances, contraceptive pills prevent the monthly development of a follicle. With no ovum to be expelled, ovulation does not occur, and therefore pregnancy cannot occur.
(b) Tubal ligation involves tying a piece of suture material around each uterine tube in two places, then cutting the tube between these two points. Sperm and eggs are thus prevented from meeting. This procedure is a surgical sterilization.
56. The uterine tubes are not attached to the ovaries and infections can exit at this area and enter the abdominal cavity.

One Last Quick Check
57. g, p. 1130
58. b, p. 1130
59. e, p. 1130
60. j, p. 1135
61. a, p. 1135
62. f, p. 1138
63. c, p. 1141
64. i, p. 1141
65. h, p. 1153
66. d, p. 1140
67. premenstrual or postovulatory
68. Prolactin
69. Oxytocin
70. meiosis
71. corpus luteum
72. Radioimmunoassay
73. Menopause
74. STDs
75. Eight
76. placenta

Diagrams
Female Pelvic Organs
1. fundus of uterus
2. uterine tube (fallopian)
3. follicle
4. fimbriae
5. endometrium
6. myometrium
7. cervical canal
8. vagina
9. cervix of uterus
10. body of uterus

Sagittal Section of Female Pelvis
1. sacral promontory
2. ureter
3. sacrouterine ligament
4. posterior cul-de-sac
5. cervix
6. fornix of vagina
7. anus
8. labium majus
9. vagina
10. labium minus
11. clitoris
12. urethra
13. symphysis pubis
14. urinary bladder
15. parietal peritoneum
16. anterior cul-de-sac
17. round ligament
18. fundus of uterus
19. body of uterus
20. ovarian ligament
21. uterine tube

CHAPTER 33

A New Human Life
1. b, p. 1162
2. b, p. 1162
3. d, p. 1162
4. a, p. 1164
5. b, p. 1167
6. a, p. 1162
7. f, p. 1162
8. t, p. 1162
9. t, p. 1164
10. f, p. 1164
11. f, p. 1164
12. f, p. 1167
13. t, p. 1164
14. t, p. 1167

Prenatal Period
15. a, p. 1169
16. b, p. 1169
17. a, p. 1169
18. b, p. 1173
19. c, p. 1179
20. t, p. 1172
21. f, p. 1169
22. f, p. 1176
23. t, p. 1169
24. t, p. 1169

Birth, or Parturition, and the

Postnatal Period
25. c, p. 1181
26. c, p. 1182
27. d, p. 1184
28. b, p. 1186
29. b, p. 1184
30. t, p. 1182
31. t, p. 1182
32. f, p. 1182
33. f, p. 1184
34. t, p. 1185

Effects of Aging
35. d, p. 1189
36. d, p. 1188
37. t, p. 1187
38. f, p. 1189

Mechanisms of Disease
39. c, p. 1191
40. a, p. 1191
41. d, p. 1192
42. b, p. 1191
43. h, p. 1192
44. f, p. 1192
45. j, p. 1191
46. g, p. 1192

Applying What You Know
47. Only about 40% of the taste buds present at age 30 remain at age 75.
48. Identical twins have the same genetic code.

One Last Quick Check
49. g, p. 1168
50. f, p. 1173
51. c, p. 1177
52. b, p. 1173

53. a, p. 1168
54. h, p. 1181
55. e, p. 1182
56. d, p. 1176
57. i, p. 1173
58. j, p. 1177
59. d, p. 1187
60. d, p. 1187
61. d, p. 1188
62. a, p. 1185
63. b, p. 1174
64. d, p. 1187
65. e, p. 1184
66. a, p. 1185
67. c, p. 1186
68. b, p. 1185

CHAPTER 34

The Science of Genetics; Chromosomes and Genes; Gene Expression
1. c, p. 1200
2. c, p. 1200
3. d, p. 1204
4. c, p. 1207
5. a, p. 1200
6. d, p. 1209
7. c, p. 1207
8. d, p. 1200
9. f, p. 1203
10. t, p. 1204
11. f, p. 1206
12. f, p. 1207
13. t, p. 1207
14. t, p. 1207
15. t, p. 1203
16. f, p. 1204

Medical Genetics; Prevention and Treatment of Genetic Diseases
17. b, p. 1209
18. b, p. 1212
19. a, p. 1213
20. c, p. 1211
21. c, p. 1213
22. b, p. 1216
23. d, pp. 1212 and 1213
24. d, p. 1220
25. c, p. 1217
26. b, p. 1217
27. f, p. 1210
28. t, p. 1206
29. f, p. 1210
30. t, p. 1216
31. t, p. 1218
32. f, p. 1210
33. t, p. 1211
34. t, p. 1217
35. t, p. 1209

Applying What You Know
36. In a form of dominance called co-dominance, the effect will be equal, causing "light brown" to occur.
37. One in four or 25%

One Last Quick Check
38. a, p. 1203
39. d, p. 1216
40. c, p. 1211
41. b, p. 1204
42. a, p. 1203
43. c, p. 1200
44. b, p. 1207
45. c, p. 1207
46. a, p. 1217
47. b, p. 1211
48. h, p. 1213
49. k, p. 1217
50. c, p. 1212
51. e, p. 1200
52. a, p. 1210
53. d, p. 1204
54. j, p. 1212
55. l, p. 1211
56. g, p. 1204

Solutions to Crossword Puzzles

CHAPTER 1

CHAPTER 2

CHAPTER 3

CHAPTER 4

CHAPTER 5

CHAPTER 6

CHAPTER 7

CHAPTER 10

CHAPTER 8

CHAPTER 11

CHAPTER 9

CHAPTER 12

CHAPTER 13

CHAPTER 16

CHAPTER 14

CHAPTER 17

CHAPTER 15

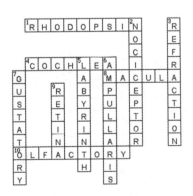

CHAPTER 18

CHAPTER 19

CHAPTER 22

CHAPTER 20

CHAPTER 23

CHAPTER 21

CHAPTER 24

CHAPTER 25

CHAPTER 28

CHAPTER 26

CHAPTER 29

CHAPTER 27

CHAPTER 30

CHAPTER 31

CHAPTER 33

CHAPTER 32

CHAPTER 34

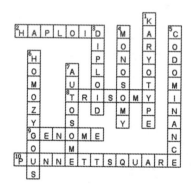

NOTES

NOTES

NOTES

NOTES

NOTES